Bumfuzzle
JUST OUT LOOKING FOR PIRATES
a sail around the world

PATRICK SCHULTE

Book Bums Publishing

Bumfuzzle
JUST OUT LOOKING FOR PIRATES
a sail around the world

_____

Cover design by WorldWide Optimize @ www.worldwide-corporate.com

Please visit Pat and Ali's website for more stories, pictures, videos, and information on their adventures. www.bumfuzzle.com

ISBN 978-0-6152-2033-8

PUBLISHED BY BOOK BUMS PUBLISHING

foreword and acknowledgments

I had never dreamed of sailing around the world. The closest I had come were daydreams of building a raft and floating down the Mississippi River, like any boy who'd ever read Tom Sawyer and grown up in the Midwest. As a boy my dad would take me to the woods to hunt deer, pheasants, or grouse. I can remember vividly the thrill of being a twelve-year-old boy walking alone through the trees with a shotgun over my shoulder. I'd read *My Side of the Mountain* and would have given anything to live in those woods and survive off the land. But at the end of the day I would climb into the car, toes frozen and stomach growling, excited to be going home.

Those sorts of adventures and dreams are for kids. By the time I graduated from high school I no longer had dreams, I had goals. Go to college, marry my beautiful high school sweetheart Ali, become a big shot trader, earn more money than my dad, own a house and a sports car, and . . .

And what? Ten years later I'd done all of that. Ali and I were young, successful, and sort of floundering. Suddenly, at only twenty-eight we had no dreams, and were realizing that the goals we had weren't necessarily what we wanted out of life.

We were fine with not having dreams. We'd come to the conclusion long ago that dreaming about something was never going to make it happen. However we were not okay with not having goals. Goals that excited us, goals that we genuinely wanted to achieve. Which is why, five years later, we are circumnavigators.

Setting out on this adventure we had another goal, to share it all with our family and friends through a website. The site that grew out of this is where much of the material for this book was lifted from. We've edited out much of my longwinded ramblings and have tried to leave a book that focuses primarily on the lengthy stretches of sailing that a circumnavigation entails, while also describing a personal side to it as well.

"The danger is that other idiots may see this story as a recipe for taking off across oceans without basic knowledge, common sense, or a well-prepared vessel." This theme was often repeated in the online cruising forum community, and was applauded by many. Well, the truth is, we hope that this book will do just that. I like to think of it as idiot encouragement. Take a chance in life. Set a goal for yourself and make it happen.

We've only got one life, and at the end of it Ali and I want our last thought to be, who is the idiot now?

We would like to say thanks to our families, and particularly to the moms. Susy, thanks for keeping Visa from closing us down while making charges in places like Eritrea, and also for keeping our life insurance up to date. At least your daughter would have been

foreword and acknowledgments

well taken care of had she ever decided to push me off the boat. A big hug goes out to my mom, who always lugged an extra suitcase around the world when visiting us. There is nothing more exciting while cruising than to open a suitcase filled with boat supplies, books, and Skittles. Also, thanks to Lorraine Burokas for her help in editing this mess. You remind me that I owe my high school English teacher an apology. And finally, a huge thank you to all of you that followed us along on this journey through our website. Nothing beat opening that e-mail inbox every day and being flooded with your support and kindness.

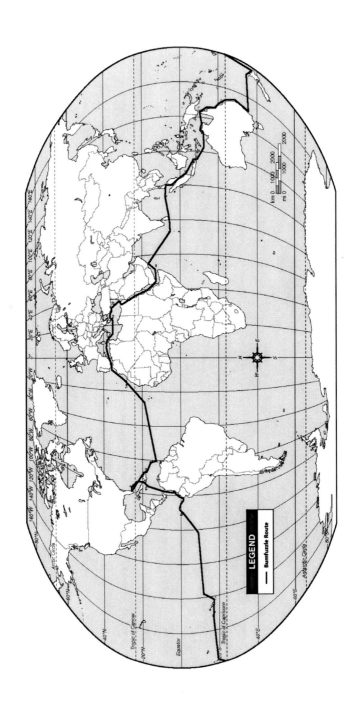

LEGEND

— Bumfuzzle Route

JUST OUT LOOKING FOR PIRATES
a sail around the world

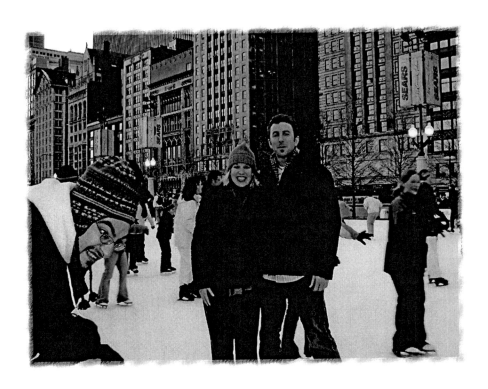

SAILING AROUND THE WORLD is not traditionally something that you are supposed to go about without first giving it some serious thought. Prevailing wisdom says that before crossing oceans on a boat you should at least be a fairly proficient coastal sailor, or barring that, should have grown up around boats and have a fair bit of knowledge as to how they work. Before buying a boat to embark on the adventure of a lifetime there should be a considerable amount of time spent researching different models, hanging out at the local docks kicking the tires, and hitching rides aboard friend's, or friends of friend's boats.

Ali and I knew all of this. I mean it's simple common sense really. And yet there we were, thinking what have we gotten ourselves into this time? Dense jungle clogged the rivers edge, where dark muddy water flowed swiftly past, as thick and undulating as a freshly poured pint of Guinness. We had arrived late the night before, unannounced and unsure if we even had permission.

Ali was awake, probably sitting on the couch reading a book, trying to relax after what had been a terrible week at sea. After peeking out the window to convince myself once again that our anchor was holding and we weren't drifting down the river aimlessly, I laid my head back down on the pillow. I hope I haven't bitten off more than I can chew I thought to myself as the sounds of this little known river on the Pacific coast of Colombia gently put me back to sleep.

JUST A YEAR OR SO earlier, Ali and I had found ourselves in the uncomfortable position of questioning what our lives were all about, what our goals for the future were. Admittedly we were both a little drunk at the time, but those types of conversations are best after a few drinks anyway. At least that's what we had always found. We'd gone through this routine before.

This particular night the conversation took an unexpected turn. While discussing our friends we realized that we were being abandoned in the city. It seemed that everybody was defecting to the suburbs, and our circle of friends who could go out on a Wednesday night on short notice had dwindled precipitously as the kids had started popping out.

We had no particular qualms with this lifestyle. We had both grown up in the suburbs of St. Paul, and at one point had even bought a suburban home ourselves. However, that little experiment only lasted nine months. We went stir crazy. Sitting in traffic twice a day staring at all the commuters with seemingly similar lives in the cars around us made us realize quickly that we had no interest in that way of life any more.

A move to Chicago solved our itchy feet for a while. We bought a condo just blocks from the Sears Tower, where Ali went to work as an administrative assistant. Meanwhile I stepped into the trading pits at the Chicago Board of Trade. We really felt our lives were perfect at that point. Being self-employed and unencumbered, I could take risks in the market that many of those around me couldn't dream of. And the risks paid off. For the next couple of years Ali paid our bills, while my trading account grew.

We drove a convertible and took three-day weekends nearly every week, cruising all over the country on short holidays to drink beer and take in a baseball or football game. Upon hearing what I did for a living, people would invariably comment, "Oh that must be stressful." But it wasn't. It was just the two of us, and we didn't have a care in the world.

And that is why that fateful night, when the conversation veered off in the direction that it did, it seemed so weird. We quickly ruled out the possibility of moving out of the city and starting a family. We wanted a family at some point, but at the time we just weren't feeling the draw.

We really needed something else though. We'd been in Chicago for over three years; and while things were great, they also felt rather ordinary. We had accomplished what we set out to do, and now we needed a new goal for ourselves.

With the commodities markets closed at 1:30, I really didn't have a whole lot to do before meeting Ali at five o'clock to walk to dinner. That led to a lot of time on the internet, where I eventually found, and became enamored of, a travel blog. It was a backpacker website and was filled with stories from around the world of people about our age experiencing the most amazing things. To my Midwestern mindset, the thought of trekking through India, camping in the Sahara, or smoking dope on a river raft in Vietnam, was completely foreign. I had also read a blog about a group of friends who had bought a sailboat and sailed around the world together. Things like this had never even crossed my mind. These people's lives were anything but ordinary.

With these thoughts burning in my mind, I suppose it was no great leap to come to the conclusion that what we really needed to do was drop everything, buy a boat, and sail off to distant lands. Of course, it's one thing to say these things late at night, belly up to the bar with a pitcher of beer in front of you. It's another thing entirely to follow through on it.

Yet that is exactly what we did. Within days deliveries of books were showing up at our door. I was consuming every bit of sailing-related material I could get my hands on. At the same time Ali was buried in envelopes and boxes, selling anything and everything we owned. She was relentless, selling off wedding gifts as easily as if they were toys from a box of cereal. If we were going to change our life, we weren't going to go about it half assed. It was all or nothing. Which, looking back now, may have contributed to our success. With no comfortable, easy life to return to it would be much harder for us to give up.

As soon as the Chicago winter let up, we hit the water. Amazingly, at this point neither of us had ever stepped foot on a sailboat in our lives. Sailing 101 would be our first taste of the cruising life. It turned out to be a less than exciting introduction. For hours, we bobbed around in a twenty-four foot monohull, practicing man overboard drills and performing one tack after another. The class lasted eight hours, and by the end we were both thoroughly bored with sailing. Had it not been for the fact that we were leaving to sail around the world in a couple of months, there is a strong possibility that would have been the last time we ever found ourselves on the water being propelled by anything other than a motor.

One thing sailing lessons taught me though, was that sailing is easy. It really is. Once I understood the fact that the sails act less like a parachute and more like an airplane wing, I figured I knew all I needed to know. I thought that as long as we understood the basic concept we could figure the rest out as we went along. Ali was with me all the way on that idea, as she had absolutely hated the class and had no desire to return for more.

Fourth of July weekend we found ourselves in Florida, where it was hot as hell. Chicago living hadn't lent itself well to getting a tan, and we looked ridiculous amongst the copper-colored denizens strolling the beaches. But it didn't matter because we were there to buy a boat. In no time at all we'd be sipping mai-tais on deserted islands. That was the plan anyway.

BEFORE ARRIVING IN FLORIDA I'd pretty much picked out our boat. It was a thirty-five foot catamaran built in France. There were three of them in the area, all in our price range, and I was sure that one of them would work out. Ali had seen the pictures I'd shown her on the internet and was as excited about seeing our new boat as I was. So when the broker led us onto the first one, we were more than a little disappointed. As we'd learn later, nearly every picture of a boat posted on the internet was taken when the boat was less than one year old. After that boats tend to look like crap. Even worse than the condition of the boat, was the layout inside. We were shocked at just how small it was, and we hardly felt comfortable at the dock inside this mini capsule. We needed to see more.

Throughout the day we looked at about ten boats, all bigger, uglier, and more expensive than the last. Finally, while walking along the dock to look at a different boat, we spotted this sparkling white image of perfection. It was thirty-five feet of superb South African engineering. We stepped aboard and knew immediately that this was our boat. It felt twice as large inside as the other boats; and it was only a year old, which meant it still looked clean and new. With our in-depth criteria satisfied we made the deal and raced back to the airport to catch an earlier flight. Our boat search and selection had lasted ten hours, and best of all had allowed us to return to Chicago for fireworks instead of sweltering in Florida.

Now that we had a boat, we had to give it a name. Superstition says it is bad luck to rename a boat, but we couldn't imagine spending the next four years explaining a name that meant absolutely nothing to us. Naming a boat is not easy. We soon had notebook pages filled with possibilities. We quickly ruled out anything with the word wind in it. As every second boat on the water either begins or ends with it. To us that would be like seeing a list of the most common baby names, picking out number one, and then bestowing that name on your child. "Yes honey, I know there are six girls in your class with the same name as you. Isn't that neat?"

When we stumbled across Bumfuzzle in an online slang dictionary we knew we had a winner. Bumfuzzle: To bewilder or confuse, used to describe something you don't understand. That pretty much summed up our feelings, and our relationship with sailing. It also had one other very important feature, its domain name was available.

From the start of all of this, we knew we wanted to share our adventure on the internet. Blogs were really in their infancy at the time, and there really wasn't a lot out there related to what we were doing. We thought that there had to be others like us out there, and telling our story might help them make the leap as well. So practically overnight we'd registered bumfuzzle.com, taught ourselves basic web design, and launched our page. Basically, this was the beginning of our trip.

FOR THE NEXT FEW WEEKS we continued to unload all of our worldly belongings for about a tenth of what they had originally cost us. We really didn't care what things sold for as long as we didn't have to store them.

Ali had quit her job a couple of months earlier in order to concentrate on our departure, while I continued to trade. As the weeks went by my trading became smaller and smaller while I tried to close out my positions. The problem was that I couldn't tell anybody what I was planning.

My business was cutthroat. In addition to being my friends, the guys I stood shoulder to shoulder with every day were also my competitors. I was in the trading pits four hours a day with one thing in mind, and that was taking everybody's money from them. Because of that I didn't think sharing the news that I was leaving to go sail around the world would be met with a party and a cake. Instead they'd try to screw me over on every trade I made.

On my last day, a Friday, I walked into the pits and told a couple of friends that I wouldn't be there on Monday. I was done, and Ali and I were going sailing. Nobody really believed me; but the talk soon circulated around the pits, and before long everybody knew. The trading floor is really a different world compared to an office job. Here the news was met almost universally by whispering behind my back, most trying to determine how much money I had really made on such and such trade, and the others predicting my demise at sea. There were no pats on the back or high fives.

When the final bell rang, I tore up my remaining trading cards and dropped them on the floor for the last time. As the pit emptied out, and I was left standing there staring up at the blinking price quotes circling the walls, one of the largest brokers in the building walked up to me. He was a nice guy whom I had stood five feet away from for three years, and made thousands of trades with, but whom I'd never really just had a talk with. It was well known by the traders that he was worth north of twenty million dollars, lived in the ritziest neighborhood, owned a bunch of outside businesses, and drove six figure cars. In these circles he was a God. He stood alongside of me, put his arm over my shoulder and said, "I wish I had done the same thing when I was your age. Now it's too late, so I just come in here and hang out with you assholes day after day."

We stood there talking for a few more minutes, and I realized that this guy whom everybody held up on a pedestal was actually filled with regrets. While everyone else was busy wishing they lived his life, he suddenly wished he could go back in time and live mine.

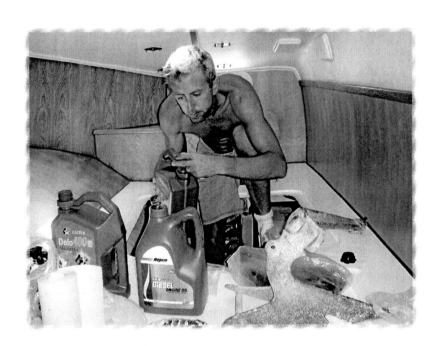

clueless at this point

THERE WERE PLENTY OF HUGS and kisses as we packed our bags and said goodbye to our families. There may have been too many. It seemed they either thought they'd see us again in a few weeks when we gave up on this stupidity, or they would never see us again. Could anybody, other than the two of us, really believe that we were saying goodbye and, see you somewhere around the world!

We really didn't have any doubt that we'd be doing exactly what we said we were going to do, sail around the world. We'd read a few books, and hell, we wouldn't be the first people to do it. Some guy had done it in 1500 something or other, and then there was that group of friends we'd read about on the internet, they'd done it too. That would make us, let's see, third? Fourth maybe?

There were doubts, but not about whether or not we could actually do it. They had much more to do with thoughts of, should we really be doing this? We're in our prime earning years. We had good jobs and a good life. Why were we leaving and throwing all of that away? Neither of us had a good answer to that. Instead we just sat quietly while those thoughts rattled around in our heads, and if pressed for an answer, we'd flippantly reply, "Why not."

And then, before we knew it, we were in Florida moving aboard a boat that we hardly knew anything about and into a lifestyle that we really knew nothing about.

SEPTEMBER 13, 2003: FORT LAUDERDALE, FLORIDA
We finally arrived in Fort Lauderdale yesterday after driving sixteen hundred miles in two days. As soon as we pulled up at the dock, we could see the guys washing our boat and putting the finishing touches on the work we had them do. She looked great.

Our boat broker was there, and he walked over to greet us. "Where's all your stuff?" he asked. That lifted our spirits a bit, as we were sure we had over packed, despite downsizing to about one percent of our former selves. I hitched a thumb over my shoulder at the boxes, just barely visible in the back of the truck.

He smiled and said, "I don't think I've ever seen a new boat owner show up without towing a trailer behind them. Good job. You don't need much to go sailing."

We spent the afternoon moving the boat from the broker's dock to our ritzy new digs at the city marina. It's a really nice place with all the facilities that anyone living on a boat could want.

We got settled in our slip without major drama. Afterwards Ali got one of the bedrooms ready while I ran to Taco Bell, and after a couple of beers we crashed. I would say it was sort of a muted celebration.

Around midnight we woke up to a strange sound on the boat, like bacon frying in a pan. I looked over the whole boat and finally gave up trying to figure out what it was. This morning while talking to our neighbor, I explained the strange noise.

He laughed as I told him about it and then cleared up the situation telling me that it was just barnacles attaching themselves to the bottom of the boat. Weird.

SEPTEMBER 23, 2003: FORT LAUDERDALE, FLORIDA
Tried to take a sail yesterday, but found once we got out of the shelter of the marina the wind was blowing twenty knots out in the ocean. That was a little much for our first sail on the boat so we turned around. Only one minor scuff as we were backing out of our slip. First one of many we are sure.

BEFORE WE MOVED ONTO THE BOAT *we told ourselves that we'd practice sailing for a couple of months before we took off for the Bahamas at the end of hurricane season. When it came right down to it though, we didn't sail a bit. Besides chickening out when we found twenty knots of wind, the only other time we left the marina was to motor along the beaches one fine, windless day. The kind of day we'd grow to both love and loath, depending on where we happened to be at the time. Loath if we were too far from our destination to motor the entire way, and love if we had enough diesel to get us there.*

The next two months turned out to be the worst two months in the history of our relationship. It seemed all we were doing was spending a lot of money on boat junk for a trip that still didn't really feel like it had begun. Day after day was spent loading the boat up with stuff that would only be necessary if we were actually at sea. It was frustrating, and a little scary to see firsthand what we had actually gotten ourselves into. We fought constantly over the most mundane things. For years I couldn't remember either of us raising our voice at the other. We had no reason to. We were stress free. Now, when it seemed we were supposed to be having fun we were instead consumed by stress. I felt like I couldn't show it though, I needed to stay strong and committed. We both kept telling ourselves, and each other, that everything would be alright once we got going. What we really needed was to get out of Florida.

But we didn't leave. Not right away. Somehow the days and weeks just continued to slip by. On the one hand, we were waiting for hurricane season to officially come to an end; but on the other hand, it was a crutch for us to lean on and an excuse to point to as to why we were still sitting there.

During this time we came to the realization that we didn't know the first thing about boats. Electronics were a mystery to me, as was plumbing and engine repair. After dropping a power cord into the water and blowing a fuse, we sat for twenty-four hours without music or lights before a friend came aboard and pointed out to me the breaker that had tripped. I'd searched for hours, it took him less than a minute. And the whole time it was right in front of me.

While I was busy realizing how little I knew about the things that make boats work, Ali was realizing just how little she knew about cooking. Trying to make out a list of foods to bring was nearly impossible. Packing flour, wheat, beans, and rice was out of the question. Neither of us had the slightest clue what to do with those things. In Chicago we'd spent four nights a week at Taco Bell, two eating our favorite pizza, and the last night at some other miscellaneous restaurant. There had never been any cooking by either of us. In the end we settled on cans. Lots and lots of cans. Campbell's soup was the big winner, followed closely by tuna, and in third place was chili. Maybe not the most well-rounded meals, but if Ali had to cook, that was as good as it was going to get.

We both had our uncertainties about the future and what this sailing thing really held in store for us; but we were in this thing deep now, and we were just going to have to work through it. When the time finally came, we just went for it.

NOVEMBER 10, 2003: BISCAYNE BAY, FLORIDA

We made it! Our first real trip was a success. We decided to leave Fort Lauderdale this morning despite some deteriorating forecasts. Seas were running about five feet with winds around twenty knots, gusting to near forty. Not an hour into the trip, I was tossing cookies over the stern rail. That was a little disconcerting, as neither of us had given much thought to the fact that we might be prone to seasickness. Fortunately Ali felt fine, and I regrouped quickly.

It took us about six hours to make the trip down to Miami and find a nice spot to anchor. We were happy to be settled in, because two hours later the winds had picked up even more and it started raining heavily. When we got into the harbor and set the anchor, I dove down on it to make sure that it was set properly and that it was completely buried in the mud. Despite the howling wind I then slept like a baby.

NOVEMBER 18, 2003: BISCAYNE BAY, FLORIDA

After a week of being stuck due to strong winds, it is finally time to leave Florida. We left very early this morning and sailed out through Stiltsville, a bunch of homes built on stilts smack dab in the middle of the reef. The winds were blowing at twenty-five knots instead of the fifteen that was forecast.

We sailed into the Gulf Stream a few miles out from land and promptly decided that today was no day to try and make it across. The waves were about eight feet and washing right over the bow, making for a very rough ride. Our port engine began smoking and we had to shut it off. Meanwhile, we had small fish being washed into the cockpit with the waves. Basically, it sucked.

After weighing our options, we decided that there was no way we would be able to make it to the Bahamas before dark, and therefore we would head back and wait for better weather for the next attempt. So what have we learned from our first two long sails? Never rush a departure date. You have to wait for a proper weather window. Besides, we aren't on a schedule, so what are we rushing around for? The forecast sucks down here though. It's supposed to be really windy for a few more days. So we wait.

AS SILLY AS IT MIGHT SOUND, after months of boat ownership, thirty miles and twenty miles were still considered long sails. We really were clueless at this point. We were getting our weather off of the evening news and were still surprised when it was incorrect. Not to mention that one of our engines was overheating and I didn't have a sniff what that might mean. Causes, effects, it was all lost on me until I pulled out the books and looked up the troubleshooting sections. Back in the harbor it would be another week before we got our second chance to cross the Gulf Stream and make it to the islands.

NOVEMBER 21, 2003: BISCAYNE BAY, FLORIDA

Still waiting. Everyone is talking about how unusual the weather has been for South Florida. We decided to get some things done on the boat as long as we are stuck here. First thing was to figure out why the engine was smoking. That was an easy one. No coolant. It was completely dry.

After that we were on to changing the oil. To empty the oil, we use a little pump to suck the oil out instead of draining it out the bottom like a car. We stick one hose into the oil and the other hose into an empty container. When I start pumping the thing, we can hear the oil going through and spitting out into the container that Ali is holding.

Then suddenly, POP! One of the hoses slipped off the fitting under the pressure of the pump. Oil blew all over the place. Ali stood there in shock, with oil dripping off her chin and splattered all over her chest. It was like a shot out of one of those biker magazines, and I have to say, it was quite sexy. I was pretty well unscathed, as the oil hose was facing the other way. When Ali came out of shock, she actually started laughing. That, of course, caught me completely off guard. Not exactly the response I expected. After we cleaned that up, we tried again, this time with a slightly larger hose that wouldn't be under so much pressure. Everything went well and now we have one engine tuned up and ready to go. Yes, just one.

NOVEMBER 25, 2003: BIMINI, BAHAMAS

At last, the Bahamas. I'll start with the crossing. We upped anchor at three a.m. in dead calm conditions. Not ideal sailing weather, though motoring across sounded good to us as long as we got there.

We repeated the previous week's departure routine, aside from one small glitch. While we motored along through Stiltsville, I saw a light in front of us. Ali was down below on the charts, directing me through the reef, so I was up top alone. The light looked like a big star sitting pretty low on the horizon.

I kept my eye on it, but for the life of me I couldn't figure out what it was. Not being a conspiracy theorist I wasn't ever under the illusion that we were being visited by a UFO, but it did seem to be coming closer. As a white outline appeared underneath the light, I suddenly realized that it was the outline of a sailboat! It took my mind a second to comprehend that we were about to T-Bone another sailboat before I spun the wheel hard over to port.

"What's going on?" Ali yelled from down at the nav station.

"Uhhh, nothing. There was a sailboat in front of us, that's all."

"What?!" Ali raced outside just in time to see the ghost ship fading back into the darkness. "Jesus Christ, watch what you're doing."

"Me? The guy was anchored right in the middle of the channel." It was a weak argument, but I had to try and defend myself somehow.

We avoid sinking two boats, motor out through the reef, and everything is going great. The seas are flat, we are making six knots, and then, disaster. Well, a small disaster anyway.

Our port engine, the same one that I had worked on just days earlier, overheated and shut down. Smoke was pouring out of the engine room. So the situation is that we have only our starboard engine. Even with the wheel cranked over to the right it can't keep us going in a straight line because of the current which is pushing us north at two knots.

We are drifting north aimlessly again, just like the week before. There is virtually no wind, so hoisting the sails won't help. I go down in the engine room, which has about fifteen cases of beer stacked up in it that have to be moved before I can access the engine. Note to self: Do not stack fifteen cases of beer above the engine again. I check the oil, and it is fine. I remove the coolant cap and it is bone freaking dry. After I fill it up again we are back on track, a little smoky smelling and nervous about our engine burning up, but otherwise okay.

Now the sun starts to come up, it is a perfect orange ball coming up over the horizon. Fifteen minutes later I am standing in the cockpit and I say to Ali, "Come on, where are all the dolphins?" half jokingly. Well, I walk up to the front of the boat, and I swear to God, there are two dolphins swimming directly in front of our bows!

I yell to Ali, and she looks at me weird, not believing me. But she comes up front anyway, sees them, and starts talking to them in their native language. The dolphins swam with us for a half hour or so, and I must say that the experience really makes you feel like they are welcoming you to their world, as corny as that might sound.

We spent the rest of the day stopping every so often to fill up the coolant. And then finally, Land Ho! We came into the cut between the North and South islands of Bimini knowing that there was only one thing we had to look out for, a shifting sandbar near the entrance.

We were tooling along nice and slow watching for the obvious shallow water and not really seeing it. And then the depth finder went, ten feet, eight, four, two and a half, "Oh crap," four feet, eight feet. Whew! Who would have guessed that we wouldn't be up on the sand when the depth finder read two point five?

After settling in, I went to customs and immigration where I paid $150 to be able to stay in their country for six months and fish all I want. We then went and celebrated with cheeseburgers and beers before heading back to the boat and collapsing into bed as the sun went down.

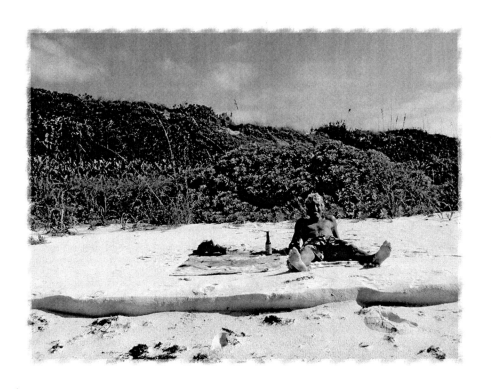

THE NEXT THREE MONTHS *flew past. Once we reached the Bahamas our lives on the boat changed quickly. When we were in the States we were under the misguided impression that we needed to get everything perfect before taking off. We needed to have four million pounds of food, one hundred cases of beer, thousands of ziplock sandwich bags (for reasons that would later completely elude us), and a whole host of other things. It was a mad rush to buy everything we could possibly ever need, because once we left we'd never have the chance again.*

It turned out that was completely wrong. The world is shrinking, and pretty much anything you can get at home you can find everywhere else.

But that wasn't the point, the point was that once we left Florida we stopped worrying. We didn't worry about anything in fact. Days and sometimes weeks went by with the two of us doing little more than reading a bunch of books, spearing a few grouper, and drinking plenty of cold beers while lying in the sun. All that stress we brought on ourselves before we left was for nothing.

Our confidence in the boat and in our ability to handle the boat grew quickly. We bounced from island to island, rarely more than a few miles apart. The ocean bottom was soft sand, nearly always under ten feet deep, and as clear as a pane of glass. Anchoring, and more importantly, anchoring securely was a breeze.

We hardly noticed the weeks slipping away, and were about as happy and carefree as two people could possibly be.

DECEMBER 2, 2003: BIMINI, BAHAMAS

It's hard to believe we are into December. It is amazing what a difference a year makes. Just about every day one of us says, "Can you believe we should be Christmas shopping?"

We have been pinned down here in Bimini for the last few days. The winds have been blowing steady at twenty knots. They're not big winds, but we are sitting tight until calmer weather appears anyway. Besides, sitting in a virtually empty bay reading books, listening to music, and soaking up the sun isn't such a bad thing.

We did get the other engine tuned up and ready to go. The whole thing took just over an hour and was completed with no oil explosion.

We have also taken to having our daily meal at around three o'clock and calling it lunner. This was done more in an effort to avoid cooking more than once a day than for any other reason. Cooking for ourselves has got to be one of the toughest things we've had to adjust to.

DECEMBER 5, 2003: GREAT HARBOR CAY, BAHAMAS

We left last night for Great Harbor Cay, an overnight sail of about eighty miles. We raised the sails, but the winds were really light and weren't much help. It was a great night to motor though, with a full moon lighting everything up for us, and not a single ship in sight.

It was a pretty uneventful trip over until I decided to throw a couple of fishing lines out. Ali started right in with the smart-ass comments, "Do you want me to start the grill now?" And, "I put out the fish fry and the tartar sauce is on the table."

So when I had a fish hit the lure and jump out of the water ten minutes later, she had to eat her words. Then when I pulled the fish up all I heard was, "He's dead isn't he?" We weren't really fishing for food at this point so I tossed him back in. Alive.

DECEMBER 9, 2003: GREAT HARBOR CAY, BAHAMAS

After a couple of weeks of windy, and decidedly cold weather, things turned around for us today. That of course prompted us to load up the dinghy with Coronas and snacks, and head over to our own private beach for a hard earned day (well maybe not too hard earned) of rest and relaxation.

DECEMBER 17, 2003: BONDS CAY, BAHAMAS

A beautiful, sunny day today. We are anchored off of Bonds Cay tonight after enjoying an absolutely perfect day. We caught a nice sized barracuda which we cooked up for dinner. Excellent. We have been seriously craving something new to eat.

DECEMBER 18, 2003: BONDS CAY, BAHAMAS

What a night. It is five a.m. and we are anxiously awaiting the sunrise. Yesterday afternoon we had a storm front roll through, bringing with it a lot of rain. It passed in about fifteen minutes. However, within the hour, the wind shifted from the south to the northwest and increased from a relatively calm fifteen knots all the way up to thirty. We had tucked in pretty close to shore to stay out of the waves generated by the south winds and now found ourselves in danger of being pushed right into the rocks. This all happened so fast that we hardly had time to think about our options.

By the time I looked at the chart searching for an alternative anchorage in which to hide from the wind, darkness had settled in. There was no safe anchorage to head to.

We decided that we had to give ourselves some more room from the rocks. Ali went to the front of the boat to raise the anchor. She looked like a sailor straight out of a movie with huge waves blasting the front of the boat and sending spray right over her head. It was pretty wild. We motored out a couple hundred yards farther from land and got the anchor to bite on the first try. We slept in shifts the rest of the night as the boat bounced and banged in the waves. We're getting out of here the minute the sun comes up.

DECEMBER 31, 2003: ROYAL ISLAND, BAHAMAS

Today we woke up to find a perfect blue sky and temps around eighty-five. What better way to spend New Year's Eve? We lounged around in the sun, I went hunting with my new spear for the first time, and we explored some old hotel ruins on the island.

We thought we were going to have this entire bay to ourselves for the night but a few boats filed in right before dark. This is the first time we've really gotten to see the beauty of a shallow draft for ourselves. Our side of the bay is only five feet deep, too shallow for the big motor boats that came in tonight, so they're all piled on top of each other in another corner far from us.

JANUARY 5, 2004: DUNMORE TOWN, BAHAMAS

We just found out that we should not have eaten that barracuda the other day as they could carry ciguatera toxin. I knew about this poisoning issue but didn't really realize it was such a big deal. Ali punched me in the arm when she found out about that. I'm sure from here on out she won't trust me when I filet some unidentifiable fish for dinner.

JANUARY 8, 2004: ROYAL ISLAND, BAHAMAS

What a day. We decided to transit the Devil's Backbone without a guide. It's a completely unmarked transit through a long section of reef that we needed to go through in order to visit Dunmore Town. We had hired a guide to bring us in and we had the route marked on the computer charts from the ride over, so I figured why pay the guy twice?

When we got out to the Backbone I was as nervous as I've ever been on our boat. The waves were rolling in about six feet high and we had to hug the coastline. I mean hug it. Like one hundred feet out from the rocks lining the shore. If we had lost an engine we would have been wrecked in a hurry. But with one eye glued to the computer, the other watching the instruments, and my hands constantly tweaking the autopilot, we made it. No problem.

While I was doing all this, Ali was sitting inside staying out of the wind where it was warm. She wasn't concerned in the least. Either she didn't realize how crazy that trip was or she just trusts me. I'm leaning towards the first one.

JANUARY 13, 2004: ALLAN'S CAY, BAHAMAS

When we arrived at our anchorage today, we found about a dozen other boats and not much room left to anchor. We were motoring around looking for a good spot, Ali at the front of the boat and me driving, when Ali suddenly asked how deep it was. I looked down to find we were in just three and a half feet, the same depth as our boat!

I tried to turn us back to deeper water but it was too late. The depth rose up more and we were aground for the first time. It was soft sand, no coral, so there was no need to panic. The only real danger was from the waves picking us up and dropping us back on the bottom.

I immediately jumped in the water, which was up to my thighs, and found that we were only about three feet away from deeper water. Ali dropped the anchor down and I walked it out fifty feet, where I set it in five feet of water. She then began cranking it back in. Within seconds *Bum* was free and floating again.

I felt pretty stupid, but later Ali told me that she was actually impressed that I knew how to get us off the sand. And in only two minutes no less. Immediately after it happened she had visions of us having to ask all the other people in the anchorage to come pull us off. Now that would have been embarrassing.

Now free, we searched around a bit more and found that just across from this crowded anchorage was a tiny cove with just enough room for one. We dropped anchor smack dab in the middle of it and now have all the space we could want.

JANUARY 17, 2004: ALLAN'S CAY, BAHAMAS
With such a nice peaceful anchorage all to ourselves we are finding it hard to come up with any reason to leave this place. Since arriving there has been plenty of sun, and virtually no wind. Not to mention the island is fun. It is teeming with wild iguanas that we've fed almost all of our bread to, nearly two loaves. And we don't even like reptiles.

JANUARY 23, 2004: NORMAN'S CAY, BAHAMAS
Wasting away the days sitting in Norman's Pond. What an incredible place to do it though. The pond is a large bay ringed almost entirely by the island, leaving only a very narrow and shallow entrance. The island was once owned by a famous drug runner and was used as his own personal paradise and refueling stop for planes bound for the U.S. from Colombia.

Right at the entrance as we were coming into the pond we'd seen a bunch of stingrays. When we went out in the dinghy later to check them out, we realized they were actually spotted eagle rays. We found them just hanging out in the shallow water, and when I dove in to check them out closer, I couldn't believe how huge they were. There was one that had a wingspan of at least eight feet. I swam down near him, stretching out my arms above him, and I wasn't even close to being as wide as he was. As he swam away his tail seemed to be at least twenty feet long. Awesome.

FEBRUARY 2, 2004: EXUMAS, BAHAMAS
I went snorkeling over to some nearby coral and within a minute I saw my first shark. My first shark while I was underwater that is. That was a bit of a rush. He didn't seem to want the two of us to get too close though, kept his distance, and appeared to be pretty harmless.

FEBUARY 6, 2004: STANIEL CAY, BAHAMAS
Today we headed over in the dinghy to Big Major Cay about a half mile away. Here we came across one of the Bahamas strangest scenes. It seems that the owners of this deserted island decided that it would be fun to put a couple pigs on it and let them run free.

Now as we approach the beach a whole herd of friendly pigs run down to greet us. They don't stop at the waters edge either, they come splashing, swimming, and snorting right out to us. It's hilarious watching as they stick their faces right into the boat. Ali was pretty brave, since she was certain that pigs don't bite, and went right to feeding them the bread we'd brought along.

FEBRUARY 22, 2004: LEE STOCKING ISLAND, BAHAMAS
Another beautiful day today. We motored down to Lee Stocking Island in the afternoon. There was just a whisper of wind, so no sailing again. Upon arriving, we found a nice little place to anchor all by ourselves.

A couple of hours later the sheep started coming in. I don't think we'll ever quite understand some cruisers. I realize that occasionally there is only a little area that is suitable for anchoring. But then there are days like today when you could anchor anywhere along this two mile stretch of island. All of it equally good. Instead of finding their own slice of beach, they feel the need to congregate like a flock of sheep. The first boat came in and anchored just off to our side. Then another boat came in and anchored directly behind us. As if that's not annoying enough, awhile later I look over at one of them and see they're staring at us through binoculars. Weirdos.

This morning when we were leaving, we passed by Rudder Cut Cay where another group of half a dozen boats were all anchored right on top of one another. Meanwhile there must have been a hundred places to anchor. I just find it weird that everybody is always saying how independent cruisers are, but instead it seems that they group up at the first chance they get. At least that's what we've found so far.

MARCH 1, 2004: GEORGE TOWN, BAHAMAS

Despite strong winds and choppy waters, we braved the long dinghy ride into town because we realized that we'd made a big mistake with immigration. We were originally given ninety days to be in the country even though you can be here for six months. The immigration officer in Bimini told us to just check in somewhere along the way and get an extension before our ninety days was up. Ninety-seven days later, we remembered.

When we found the office, we opened the door and walked right in. The room was barely large enough for a desk. The immigration officer looked up at us and said, "You don't knock?"

Oops, that wasn't a good start. The office was in a large government building, and we'd assumed that behind the door would be a good sized office with a receptionist. Wrong. She told us to sit outside and wait.

She let us sweat it out for a while before calling us in. When we told her we were looking for an extension, she asked to see our paperwork. After about two seconds she realized that we were a week overdue. She didn't seem too happy, but gave us the paperwork to fill out and then informed us that the extension officer would be in on Wednesday morning. She made it pretty clear that we are to be waiting outside the office at nine o'clock sharp. So now we are just hoping that they go easy on us and let us stay in the country another six weeks. Otherwise, I'm not sure what we will have to do. We certainly can't head over to Haiti!

MARCH 3, 2004: GEORGE TOWN, BAHAMAS

We just got done with the immigration office. We made sure we were waiting outside the office ten minutes early dressed in our cleanest shirts. When the lady we'd spoken to the other day arrived, she looked at us and said, "You are a day late aren't you?"

We told her that we were sure she said Wednesday. She just looked down her nose at us and went into the office. Awhile later we were called in, given a little scolding by the extension officer, then granted an additional forty-five days.

The whole thing was kind of funny. It felt just like when I was a little kid at school and would get sent down to the principal's office. All that nervous apprehension.

MARCH 16, 2004: GEORGE TOWN, BAHAMAS

After nearly three weeks, we are finally getting prepared to get out of here. We've had a great time in George Town but are definitely ready to get out of the hustle and bustle.

We lived in Chicago, and now we consider this hustle and bustle. It's funny how much our outlook has changed. In fact, we just realized that we have been living on the boat for six months. It's starting to feel as if this trip is going to fly by.

MARCH 18, 2004: GEORGE TOWN, BAHAMAS

Sorry Ali. Today I committed the ultimate rookie sailor mistake and it almost cost us our boat. It started last night with a crappy night of sleep due to a wind shift right after we went to bed. The waves made the boat really loud and uncomfortable. So right out of the chute this morning, we were tired.

We upped anchor bright and early with the wind direction way off from where it was supposed to have been according to the previous morning's forecast. It was blowing about fifteen knots in the harbor, and I figured it wouldn't be that bad, although I knew our chances of doing much sailing weren't looking good.

The wind direction was about thirty degrees off the bow, which is right at our limit as far as putting up a sail, so we just fired up the engines and motored out. An hour later we were breaking out of the harbor into the open ocean. Here the wind was howling at close to twenty-five knots. This is the point for which I owe Ali an apology. She asked me if I thought it was still worth going today, or if we should just turn around and anchor at a nearby spot. I told her to make a decision, even though I knew full well that she wanted to stop and anchor. When she didn't. I said, "Fine, we'll turn around." Knowing, of course, by the tone I used that she wouldn't let me turn around. For some reason I was determined to get out of George Town today. Big mistake.

Conditions didn't seem that bad at first. We were able to put up the jib and motorsail close to the wind. There was even another catamaran behind us doing the same thing. We continued on in these conditions for ten miles and now needed to turn east for a two-hour stretch through some coral heads. The problem was that it would be dead on to the wind. By now the waves were about eight feet. We turned east, pounding into the waves for a couple of miles before the trouble started.

First our port engine overheated, bringing flashbacks of the last time it had happened in the Gulf Stream under very similar circumstances. Then, with only the starboard engine trying to power us through these big waves, it too overheated and shut down. We decided since the water was only ten feet deep to just drop the anchor. This kept us pointed into the waves and stopped us from losing valuable miles floating backwards while I worked on getting the engines going again.

While I anchored, Ali went below and started clearing out the engine rooms, but not before first pointing out that the two fishing lines we had been trolling had floated underneath the boat. I tried pulling them in, but couldn't get them loose and was afraid they would get all tangled up in the props. I dove in the water with the boat slamming up and down in the waves, and sure enough both lines were wrapped in the prop. With the waves flowing under the boat that fast, the prop had kept spinning slowly even though it was in neutral, and both lines were twisting themselves around and around. I dove under once to try to untangle them but knew right away I had no chance, I was afraid the boat would lift up and slam down on top of me. Ali handed me the dive knife and I dove under one more time to cut the lines free. One problem taken care of.

When we checked the engines, we found the port engine was completely out of coolant. My first thought was that the raw water pump's impeller was shot, but there was virtually no way to replace it right now. The engine was too hot and we were rocking too much. The other engine seemed fine, just hot. I topped off the coolant and made the decision to turn around and tuck into an anchorage that was shown on the charts just two miles behind us.

We quickly made our way back and turned into the anchorage. Unfortunately, the anchorage wasn't protected from the rough conditions. In fact, it was nothing more than a few large boulders enclosing a long narrow bay and not doing much to knock down the worst of the weather. However, with our choices severely limited, we decided to give it a try.

It was nearly a half-mile motor from the entrance of the bay to the anchorage area, and we made our way through as slowly and carefully as we could. Beeeeep! Suddenly the port engine overheated and shut down again, leaving us in a precarious position, surrounded by rocks and rough seas with just one unreliable engine.

It seemed like things were looking up as we somehow managed to get to the anchorage area. As soon as we did, I jumped in the water to make sure the anchor set, and just about started crying when I saw the ocean floor. It was solid rock. For the first time in the Bahamas there was no sand at all, just a few scattered, very small coral heads sitting on top of a hard packed floor.

I was desperately trying to get the anchor jammed up against some coral as the boat drifted quickly backwards. Meanwhile, Ali was frantically dropping more chain in an effort to buy me a few more seconds to work with. It seemed futile as I was dragged along underwater. There was simply no soft bottom anywhere.

Finally, with the boat a mere thirty yards from the rocks, we got it stopped. Though it was less than secure, with the anchor just laying on its side wedged against a small piece of coral. I got back on the boat and refilled the coolant while Ali kept watch to make sure we weren't dragging. We got the engine going and pulled forward again. Not sure what else to do, and wanting nothing more than to get the boat anchored, we dropped the anchor and tried again. I jumped in and kept searching for anything to stick the anchor into, but this time I couldn't find anything at all. We knew we were in about the worst possible position we could be in at this point.

There was no choice but to get back out into open water. At least out there we could raise the sails and not be forced to rely on our overheating engines to keep us out of danger. Somehow we managed to inch our way back out of the "anchorage" without overheating an engine, and at last we found ourselves in the relative safety of the large breaking seas.

At this point there was no place to anchor to the south, we couldn't go east because that's where the wind and waves were, and we couldn't go west because it was all islands and rocks. That left only the direction we had come from. The only choice was to go back to George Town with our tails between our legs. The bright side was that we were able to shut off the engines and sail there.

Three hours later we limped back into George Town. We had spent nine hours getting our asses kicked, and nearly destroyed our boat, all so we could return to where we had been anchored that morning. Ali had, of course, been upset by all of this, but the minute the anchor was set and we were safe she was her old self again. We cleaned up the boat, Ali cooked dinner, and I worked on the engines. It almost felt like the day hadn't even happened, except that we were sore, bruised, cut up, and exhausted.

Sitting here now, I can't believe that we didn't lose our boat today. We made every stupid mistake you can make. The biggest mistake, of course, was going out in terrible weather for absolutely no reason except that we were bored with George Town and wanted to move on.

MARCH 22, 2004: SALT POND, BAHAMAS
An absolutely beautiful day today. Great for sailing too, especially compared to our bungling misadventure the other day. When we arrived we anchored, cleaned up the boat, had a few beers, dinner, and watched the sun go down on a very good day.

MARCH 28, 2004: SALT POND, BAHAMAS
Yesterday we woke to find that our water pressure pump wasn't working. We had an extra one onboard, so I thought I would just switch them out. I unscrewed the old one, tipped it over and then back upright. Ta-dah! Somehow it's working like new again. Screwed it back in and I was done. Yes, I am quite the mechanic. Now what else can I fix?

MARCH 31, 2004: EN ROUTE TO ACKINS ISLAND
We upped anchor this morning with no wind. The wind sensor thingymabob actually showed 0.0 knots. There are supposed to be light winds for a few days, which should work out okay since we are headed for an island 120 miles away, our longest straight shot so far.

Twelve hours later and the wind has remained incredibly calm all day. We have been motoring the entire time, alternating between the engines two hours at a time.

We had a couple of dolphins come by, though they didn't get too close. Aside from that, it was a pretty uneventful afternoon. One cool thing about the day was how the blue of the sky matched the still water perfectly. There were times when we would look out at the water and could not see the horizon at all. The two blended together so perfectly that it was like a blue wall started fifty feet away from the boat and went on infinitely. As if we were motoring through the sky.

APRIL 7, 2004: MATTHEW TOWN, BAHAMAS
After a week in Matthew Town, all of our preparations are done and we are ready to go. We filled the gas tanks, bought a few groceries, went up the mast a couple of times to fix the lights, called home, and cleared ourselves out of the country. We're set to go tomorrow. Our first real passage.

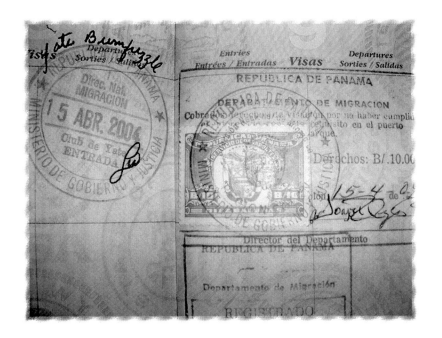

Visas Departures
Sorties / Salidas

Entries   Departures
Entrées / Entradas **Visas** Sorties / Salidas

REPUBLICA DE PANAMA

DEPARTAMENTO DE MIGRACION

Cobro de pasaporte visado por no haber cumplido
el requisito en el puerto

Derechos: B/.10.00

15-4 de

Director del Departamento

REPUBLICA DE PANAMA

Departamento de Migración

REGISTRADO

Direc. Nal.
MIGRACION

15 ABR. 2004

Club de Yate
ENTRADA

MINISTERIO DE GOBIERNO Y JUSTICIA

I will go alone

APRIL 8, 2004: EN ROUTE TO PANAMA

We left this morning for Panama. It finally feels like a true adventure now. The Bahamas were like putting training wheels on a ten-year-old kid's bike. Sure, he could still wipe out, but it's not very likely that he'll hurt himself. Try as we might, we just couldn't wreck our boat in the Bahamas. The place is simply too idiot proof.

Now we are truly out here in the middle of nowhere with no nice safe anchorages to tuck into when the weather gets ugly. For the first time, this sailing thing is really exciting. Not an easy feat to accomplish while moving at the pace of a slow jog.

Right now we are passing about six miles off the coast of Cuba on our way through the Windward Passage. After seeing only two ships all day, as soon as it got dark three more popped up on the radar screen. The nice thing along this stretch is that there are specific shipping lanes running north and south. We tucked into the southbound lane as close to the edge as we could. So far all the ships have been on the same course as us but passing at a safe distance off to our side. I guess the only real concern right now would be to have one bear right down on us from behind. What are the chances of that though?

APRIL 9, 2004: EN ROUTE TO PANAMA

Today went from very light winds to absolutely no wind at all. Here we are smack dab in the middle of Cuba, Haiti, and Jamaica, in an area called the Windward Passage, and we are completely becalmed. The one upside to this is that dolphins seem to love it when we are motoring slowly.

Twice today we were visited by spotted dolphins. The first group this morning came by and swam along with us for about five minutes. Then right before sundown a couple dozen came by to put on a show. These guys were jumping all the way out of the water and zooming from one side of the boat to the other. They always make our day; and since this was the first time we had ever seen these little ones, it was even more fun.

As of right now we are making some pretty slow progress and are already doing the calculations to see what speed we would have to average to get there by a certain number of days. Not much we can do about it though, so it's not really worth worrying about. The first day we made just ninety-two miles out of the trip's 800. Today doesn't look like it will match even that paltry number.

APRIL 11, 2004: EN ROUTE TO PANAMA

Two a.m. It's been three days now, and the wind has yet to give us much help. We are averaging just ninety miles a day, or less than four knots per hour. That is way slower than we anticipated and we're now looking at a nine-day passage. We did sail all day yesterday which was nice, even if it was at only three knots.

Late last night we had dolphins show up. It was really cool watching them leave a bioluminescent trail of green behind them as they swam. It would be nice if that became a nightly occurrence.

We are still hoping for more wind. It seems like the forecast just keeps pushing it a little bit farther south. Eventually we should catch up with some.

TWELVE HOURS LATER now and still no wind. It has hardly even blown enough to make our little U.S. flag flap. Right now we are motoring, trying to get south. On the weather maps it looks like there might be wind about a day's motor south of us. Normally, we would be able to motorsail, but right now when we motor we outrun the wind and the sail ends up flapping limply in the breeze. We have tried about every sail combination we can think of in an effort to squeeze out an extra half knot, but with no results. It's going to be a long passage.

APRIL 12, 2004: EN ROUTE TO PANAMA

What a difference a day makes. Last night the wind finally began to pick up. We hoisted the main and the screecher, and within an hour we were cruising along at six knots. The wind continued to build and by early morning we knew we should have taken the screecher down earlier. That sail is for light winds and here we were flying along with wind well over twenty knots. When we tried furling it, we couldn't get it to wrap up because of the strong wind. It took us four attempts before we got it to roll in, all the while the boat was swerving all over the place. After much swearing and yelling the ordeal was over, with promises that we would get the sail in sooner next time.

We put out the jib and cruised along nicely after that. The wind has stayed with us all day and we've continued to average over seven knots. Maybe we'll make it to Panama in six days after all. We were starting to worry that we would never get the boat moving. We've read that we should be able to sail at half of the wind speed. That seems pretty ambitious, but we were starting to wonder if we were moving so slow because of our lack of sailing skills or if there was a problem with the boat. I think we have already established that there are no sailing skills onboard, but we can chalk this one up to just a lack of wind.

Last night we had a lot of ship traffic. Ali woke up at one point to find me swerving between three container ships. I had been in contact with one of the ships that seemed to be coming right up on us from behind. We talked for a minute and he altered course to give us a little more room. However the other two ships seemed determined to run us down, and I ended up having to alter course forty degrees at the last minute to slide behind them. It can get confusing out here in the dark with nothing to go by but a couple of colored lights.

Later on in the night, Ali woke me up to ask about a ship that was headed right for us. She had already altered course to make sure we would steer safely by him, but now she wanted my reassurance. Of course when I came up I was still half asleep and thought the ship was going the opposite direction of what it actually was. I promptly scared the crap out of both of us.

"Jesus, turn right!"

"What? Seriously?" Ali yelled.

"Hurry up, turn thirty degrees," I said. Ali complied, but seemed confused, and began explaining the presence of the green running light and the lack of a red one.

"Shit! Turn left. A lot!" I screamed, as what she was saying finally clicked in my groggy mind. A minute later we were slipping behind a passing ship, far too close for comfort. We decided that from now on whoever was awake would have to be the final judge. It seems we are having to make a lot of new rules for ourselves.

APRIL 13, 2004: EN ROUTE TO PANAMA

"Pat! There's a ton of water in here." For some reason those words are spoken all too often. This time the water was in the bathroom and was overflowing the bilge. Luckily, or possibly not, it wasn't a thru-hull. It was, unfortunately, all of our freshwater. The freshwater feed for the watermaker had somehow slipped its fitting and had promptly emptied the contents of our freshwater tanks. All 140 gallons.

After getting the water mopped up and refitting the hose, we fired up the watermaker to make more water. All we got was an alarm. I tried everything, but couldn't get it to start up. So with 200 miles to go we've got about two gallons of freshwater left.

APRIL 14, 2004: EN ROUTE TO PANAMA

Right now I'm sitting on the couch watching the waves pick up the boat. We then surf down the front at seven knots before sliding back into the trough and slowing to four knots. Nice and peaceful, like a grandfather clock. And with under a day to go, we are getting excited.

I can hardly believe that we took our eight hours of sailing lessons a year ago on Lake Michigan. Now here we are about to complete a one-week open ocean passage. I'll bet there are a lot of people who have been sailing their whole lives who have never been on a passage this long. I'm feeling pretty pleased with the two of us. Out of all the cruisers we met in the Bahamas this year, we didn't meet one other boat that was going this way. And the looks we got when we told them what we were doing, it was like they wanted to have us committed to the insane asylum. Yet here we are.

APRIL 15, 2004: COLÓN, PANAMA

We made it. Seven days on the dot. What a great feeling it was to drop the anchor.

As we made our final approach this morning, we had to slow down and wait for the sun to come up, since all we could see in the darkness were hundreds of lights from the ships anchored all over the place. To try and pick our way through there in the dark would have been crazy. Needless to say, the three hours or so that we were bobbing around waiting for light lasted forever. Eventually though we were able to weave our way between the dozens of container ships that were anchored out waiting for their turn to transit the canal.

As soon as we got in, I headed ashore to start the customs and immigration process. They weren't open yet, and I was told to come back in the afternoon. So I filled up our water jug and headed back to the boat. I thought that having more water in the tank might make the watermaker work. It didn't.

Completely confused, I sat down and went through the steps one by one. It didn't take long before I figured out the problem. I hadn't reopened the seacock for the saltwater feed to the pump. It's kind of hard to make freshwater out of seawater if you don't add the seawater first. Problem solved. Ali rolled her eyes at me and then got right to work cleaning the boat, doing dishes that had piled up, and getting the salt off of everything.

Next it was back to shore to see about immigration. I spent an hour or so with the people there and got a stamp in our passports. But that was just the beginning. The rest of the afternoon was spent running from one office to another filling out paperwork that would then be filed in towering boxes lined up against the walls. A computerized system seemed about as far off in the future as George Jetson's flying car.

Back at the yacht club, we finally got to do what had been on our minds all day long, eat something that we hadn't warmed up out of a can. It was clear, from the prices alone, that we were a long way from home. In the Bahamas everything had cost 20% more than at home, here it was a 75% discount. I'm sure our waitress had no idea why we were so happy when she gave us our bill.

Ali and I were discussing the passage today and decided that we did pretty damn good. Out of 810 miles we had managed to sail the boat without engines for over 670 of them. We didn't eat very well, which we think we will be able to improve on a little bit next time, now that we have a feel for what it is like out there for that long. We slept pretty well after we got used to our shift schedule. There were some times that we were just super tired of being out there, but there were also times that we just sat and enjoyed the immensity of the whole thing. Overall it really wasn't too bad, and we aren't dreading the next big passage, which is what I was afraid was going to happen.

APRIL 25, 2004: COLÓN, PANAMA
After ten days in Panama, tomorrow is the big day. We are scheduled to transit the Panama Canal at 4:30 in the morning. That is about the best time we could get, since the earlier we get started the better our chances are of making it through in one day. At the bar, we rustled up the necessary line handlers and it looks like we're ready to go.

APRIL 26, 2004: COLÓN, PANAMA
Delayed! We woke up at four in the morning to wait for our pilot and begin our transit. Around six o'clock we finally got the call over the VHF telling us that it wasn't going to happen today. We were told to call back later to find out what time we'd be going tomorrow. No explanation given as to why we were cancelled.

APRIL 27, 2004: BALBOA, PANAMA
The Pacific Ocean, how very cool. After yesterday's fiasco we were really hoping for better luck today, and we got it. Our pilot showed up promptly at 4:30 and we were underway. Actually they make it very clear that they aren't pilots, they are advisors. It must help to avoid litigation, I suppose.

There were three sailboats going through this morning. Since we were the widest and sturdiest boat, they tied us up side by side, with *Bum* in the middle. It was fine by me as it meant that we didn't have to do any of the line handling. A lot of cruisers make a big deal about how they are going to be tied up in the locks, but frankly, I don't see what the fuss is all about. It isn't complicated and there didn't seem to be any stress on the boats.

We were up and through the first set of locks by eight o'clock. We motored across the muddy brown waters of Gatun Lake for a few hours, and were at the down locks by noon.

By now a big seventy-foot sailboat had caught up with us, and also a small boat that hadn't made it through the day before. The seventy footer apparently had an owner on it who fancied himself a big shot famous sailor. Anyway, upon arriving at these locks we were told we would go in two rows. Three boats in one line and two in the other. However Mr. Big Shot had another plan and actually had the gall to say, "Why don't we tie up those four *small* boats together and I will go alone." What a wanker. Four boats tied up side by side, yeah, that would work. Eventually they agreed to do three rows and he got to go by himself after all.

By early afternoon we had exited the last lock and entered the Pacific Ocean. I was saying to Ali how cool I thought it was and how this is one of those unique life experiences not many people get to do. Her response was that she was just glad to be out of Colón. I tell you, nothing impresses this girl.

OUR FEW SHORT WEEKS in Panama were fully consumed with transiting the canal, filling out copious amounts of bureaucratic paperwork (twenty-two crew lists in all), and preparing for the next leg of the journey, the Pacific crossing.

As part of those preparations, we had the boat hauled out and the bottom painted. It hadn't been done since the boat was new, and we were growing some long grass in the tropical water. With thousands of miles of blue water in front of us we wanted to be slicing through it like a hot knife through butter.

The haulout is when we first noticed some major problems with the boat. There were a couple of big bubbles just under the waterline. I could press down a full inch before they popped backed out again, like pressing in on a plastic water bottle. I didn't know what exactly that meant until later when I did a little research on the internet. It was not good news. It looked like we had delamination issues.

We sent out a few e-mails to our surveyor and the boat manufacturer, but basically got the run around and denials of any responsibility. It was clear from their tone that neither of them wanted anything to do with a delaminated boat.

We decided that Panama didn't seem like the best place to get the boat fixed, with what seemed to be a lack of professionals in that line of work. Instead we finished painting, plopped her back in the water, and headed west. If Bum could just hold together another six months we could fix her up in New Zealand. If not, well who knows.

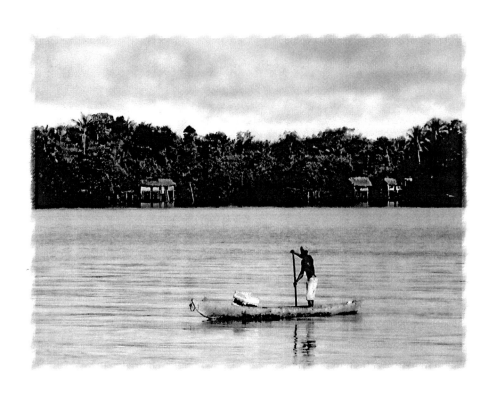

suspicious looking Colombians

GETTING READY FOR THE ROUGHLY *four thousand miles of Pacific Ocean in front of us was a lot less daunting than I would have expected. After the Panama crossing, our confidence was higher than ever. Neither one of us was the least bit concerned by what should have seemed a monumental undertaking. We just went about our business, doing the typical grocery shopping and filling up of diesel, while not giving a whole lot of thought or discussion to what lay ahead of us. The day we left you couldn't have distinguished by the attitude on the boat whether we were leaving to sail ten miles or a thousand.*

MAY 14, 2004: EN ROUTE TO GALAPAGOS ISLANDS

We left yesterday morning for the Galapagos. So far it has been an incredibly boring slow trip, though we did have a lot of dolphins around us yesterday. They didn't spend much time in our bow wave like they usually do, but they were a lot more active than we normally see. There were more than a hundred of them at one point, all very playful and making a lot of big jumps. The little ones especially were getting some huge air.

We managed to motorsail a total of 120 miles on the day. The entire trip is about 940. The actual distance as the crow flies is a lot less than that, but conventional wisdom says to get south while you can before heading west to the islands. This is because of the prevailing winds which are from the southeast to southwest.

MAY 18, 2004: BUENAVENTURA, COLOMBIA

Four days later now, and I'm not sure just what the hell happened, but here we are in Colombia. On our second night out, we were still making some decent progress motorsailing south. The forecast for the next day showed light headwinds, but I figured if we could motor through it and get in one more day of heading south, then we should be able to turn west towards the Galapagos.

Unfortunately when the wind showed up, it was twenty-five knots and was out of the southwest, the direction we needed to go. Instead we were forced to sail southeast directly towards the coast of South America. For some reason while sailing this direction, we couldn't get the sails balanced correctly to save our lives. Eventually we gave up and ran an engine to help keep us going straight, even if it was the wrong direction.

Throughout the day the winds continued to blow and the seas kept getting bigger, eventually topping out at twelve feet. I really have no idea how to judge wave heights, but guessed this by the fact that they were well over my head while standing on deck. Compounding our problem with trying to sail into the growing weather was the Humboldt Current running north along the coast at up to two knots. We weren't making any headway, and in fact were only getting farther and farther away from the Galapagos Islands.

By dark we were way off course, over one hundred miles east of where we wanted to be. The winds had kicked up to over thirty knots now and the seas had grown proportionately. Wind, waves, and current were all having their way with us. We were having to run an engine just to keep ourselves from moving 180 degrees in the wrong direction and were burning a lot of fuel. Smashing headlong into the waves was taking its toll on us; and after three days, we were exhausted.

The next day we were less than twenty-four hours off the coast of Colombia and moving farther away from our destination by the hour. We needed a new plan, and by that afternoon we finally came up with one. Turn the boat downwind and visit Colombia.

Our charts showed a large river, and fourteen miles up was the town of Bueneventura. All we wanted to do was anchor, sleep, and top off our diesel before making another run at the Pacific.

It felt great to turn the boat downwind and stop battling the waves. We had an easy sail overnight, and by late afternoon we were at the river. Unfortunately our timing was off and we caught the outgoing tide, making for an extremely slow motor up the deserted, but well-marked river. Around midnight we dropped our anchor in the murky, fast-moving water. The anchor grabbed, and within minutes we were both sound asleep.

COLOMBIA WAS A TRIP. *We honestly had no idea what to expect when we arrived, and weren't sure if we'd be welcomed or locked up. First thing in the morning a boat came by and picked me up, the man inside saying that I needed to see the port captain.*

It became clear pretty quickly that the officials had never seen a pleasure boat in Bueneventura before. At the office everybody came by to have a look at me and say hola, but in the end the port captain refused to deal with me. It seemed to be because I spoke about twenty words of Spanish and he and the rest of the office combined could speak three words of English. We were getting nowhere.

I was soon pawned off on an unsuspecting young guy who spoke excellent English and worked for a shipping agency there in the port. He was thrilled to get the chance to work with me and practice his English. For the next few hours, we zipped around town in the rain on a moped. Our agent gave me his poncho so that all that was visible was my big white head. We drew all sorts of attention as we drove down the streets, with every person we passed stopping to turn and stare. By the time we wrapped up all the paperwork and he dropped me off at the dock, it seemed the entire city knew of our arrival.

At the dock I found about a hundred spectators gathered around, just watching our boat sit at anchor fifty yards away in the middle of the river. I tracked down the boat taxi guy who offered me a ride out to Bum for twenty dollars. That was a ludicrous amount. A more reasonable price would have been twenty cents. I tried negotiating with him, which the gathered crowd enjoyed immensely, but he wasn't budging. Finally I mimed that I was going to jump in the water and swim out to the boat. That made everybody laugh, including the driver, and he finally agreed on five dollars, which included bringing out the customs officials later on.

Over the next couple of days Ali and I wandered around town, constantly garnering a lot of attention along the way. We had fun with it, though. One boy followed us for so long that we eventually bought him a Coke and a slice of pizza. I'll never forget the grin on his face.

We actually had a hard time spending the roughly forty U.S. dollars we had gotten out of the ATM. Everything was so cheap it was ridiculous. At the bakery we loaded up with more bread, cookies, and donuts than we could possibly need and walked away only two dollars lighter.

This was the first time we'd ever been somewhere that we looked so out of place. It was a little unnerving at first, but we soon realized that everybody was happy to see us, and to have us there visiting their hometown.

AFTER A FEW DAYS *the forecast looked a little more promising, and we prepared the boat, getting ready for an early morning departure.*

MAY 20, 2004: EN ROUTE TO GALAPAGOS . . . AGAIN

Around three a.m. last night I heard a strange noise. After living on the boat for a few months we've both become acutely attuned to her noises. I can tell if a drop of water came from the kitchen sink or off of the standing rigging and if a slight bump outside was just a branch floating down the river or something more ominous.

This time the bump didn't strike me as a normal boat noise, so I lifted my groggy head and took a look out the window at the foot of the bed. Staring right back at me was a boatload of very suspicious looking Colombians. Next thing I knew, there were feet scrambling by and jumping into the boat. Ali and I leaped out of bed.

"You're naked!" she yelled.

Oh yeah. Crap. I reached for my boxers and followed her out one nude step behind.

By the time we got outside, their boat was already backing up quickly while the five guys inside kept repeating, "No problem, no problem, *Policia.*"

We were yelling back at them, though unfortunately we don't know any good cuss words in Spanish. We were saying, "No *Policia*," as they kept trying to convince us they were the police while at the same time spinning around and speeding off.

Once they were gone, we grabbed a flashlight to have a look around, even though we were sure there was nothing lying about for them to take. It didn't take long to figure out what they had been doing. The outboard motor lock was broken. Actually not the lock itself, but one of the motor handles that the padlock goes through. Our thief must have realized he made too much noise when he broke that and was spooked.

It's kind of funny that they would have even attempted to steal the motor. Aside from the padlock, the outboard was also tied at the bottom to keep it from swinging, which I doubt anybody would have noticed in the dark. Then there is the fact that the motor sits directly above our cabin, and no matter how good a thief you are, you cannot sneak around on a boat carrying a motor without being heard. Also, the outboard is really heavy, and the mount that it is on is pretty high. I am 6'2" and have a hard time lifting it up high enough to get it off. So unless this guy was pretty tall, or Popeye, I don't think the motor was going anywhere, even if he had gotten it undone.

Funny thing about the whole incident was that we weren't even upset about it, nor did it even get our adrenaline going. Really it was such a pathetic attempt that the whole thing was laughable. In fact we were so unaffected that we just went right back to bed.

This morning we upped anchor and headed down the river. It was a much quicker ride on the way, out and before we knew it we were back in the ocean and on our way to the Galapagos again. At least we hope we're on our way to the Galapagos this time.

MAY 22, 2004: EN ROUTE TO GALAPAGOS ISLANDS
It is only day three of the passage, and we are ready to go insane. The passage from Panama to the Galapagos has to be one of the worst there is. The wind never stops blowing from the direction of the islands, and so here we are still pinned along the coast of South America. I'm not sure how we are ever going to get this boat pointed in the right direction. The frustration level is at an all time high.

MAY 24, 2004: EN ROUTE TO GALAPAGOS ISLANDS
It is day five, and for the first time since leaving Panama, we are pointing westward. Actually northwest, which if we continued to sail would put us hundreds of miles north of the Galapagos. We are hopeful that the wind will shift a bit more and we'll get things straightened out. We've got five hundred miles straight west to go.

We had a line break today. It is the line that runs from the top of the mast to the back of the boom. I am sure it has a name, but I don't know what it is. It snapped right in the middle, so now there is about twenty-five feet of line flailing around at the top of the mast. I rigged the spare halyard to replace it for the time being. Neither of us is really sure if that line was used to actually support the boom or just to help adjust it, but the backup plan seems to work fine for now.

MAY 25, 2004: EN ROUTE TO GALAPAGOS ISLANDS
This morning while I was sleeping, Ali went outside and was surprised by a small boat with an outboard engine and three guys on it. Being two hundred miles from land, it seemed an unlikely place to see an open fishing boat full of men, but they simply waved and moved on.

Later in the day with strong winds and pretty big seas, another small boat appeared out of the trough of a wave. They were waving and pointing for us to turn. Problem was that they wanted us to turn right into the wind. That wasn't going to work, so I just turned as much as I could. A minute later we sailed right over their net lines, which they then promptly got their own prop wrapped up in. We continued past them while keeping a sharp eye out for more nets.

A few minutes later a string of buoys lined the horizon. There was no getting around them, so we tried to sail between them instead. This time we got snagged though, and we were soon dragging a long line of nets behind the boat. I didn't really know what to do other than drop our sails and dive in the water to unhook us. But with winds at twenty knots jumping in the water with a bunch of fishing nets seemed like a bad idea.

Instead I grabbed the dive knife, reached under the water and cut the line. Problem solved. A few minutes later a little boat appeared alongside of us. The guy on the front was holding a green line like the one I had just cut, and he was making a slicing motion across it. It was quite obvious what he was trying to say, but I decided to just play dumb by pointing in front of us like I was asking which way to go. They eventually got tired of this and moved off. With miles of nets, I am sure one cut didn't sink the whole thing, and it would just require a little repairing. I felt bad about it, but still don't see what the other option was. It seems like a risk that those guys take when they cover the ocean with nets as far as the eye can see.

MAY 26, 2004: EN ROUTE TO GALAPAGOS ISLANDS
I just realized that since we left for the Galapagos two weeks ago not once have we actually had the boat pointed towards them, not even within thirty degrees of them. That's bad.

As we have been doing the entire passage, we are currently beating into big seas and not headed towards our intended landfall. It is passages like this that makes us think that maybe driving around the world, an option we briefly considered, might not have been such a bad idea. I mean, we will have wasted over two weeks of our lives to travel just nine hundred miles. A person could walk that distance in less time. Anyway, our spirits are down right now, but not out just yet. We'll keep our fingers crossed that tomorrow's forecast is right for once.

MAY 28, 2004: EN ROUTE TO GALAPAGOS ISLANDS
We are giddy with the anticipation of landfall tomorrow morning. Knowing that this is the last night of the passage is a terrific feeling.

When we left Colombia, we raised the mainsail and the jib. Since then, nine days ago, we have not made one change. The track on our charts shows a straight line south out of Colombia and then a big tack pointing us back to the north. After that we just followed the slowly changing direction of the wind. Our line makes a very gradual arc looping well north of the Galapagos in the middle and then right down to the islands at the end.

MAY 30, 2004: ISLA SANTA CRUZ, GALAPAGOS
Land Freakin' Ho! And after sailing 1450 miles to cover just 900, it's about time. A host of problems greeted us as we made our way into Academy Bay. First we found we had another burst water line and had an engine compartment full of our freshwater. Then as we dropped the anchor, our windlass jammed up, blowing a fuse. There seemed to be no end to this passage. Fortunately when I finally went ashore, I found the port officials to be extremely friendly and welcoming. In no time I had secured our twenty day visa and we were free to enjoy the island.

We went ashore and downed a few well-earned *cervezas* with cheap steaks and fried plantains. By seven o'clock we were back on the boat sound asleep for twelve hours of uninterrupted sleep.

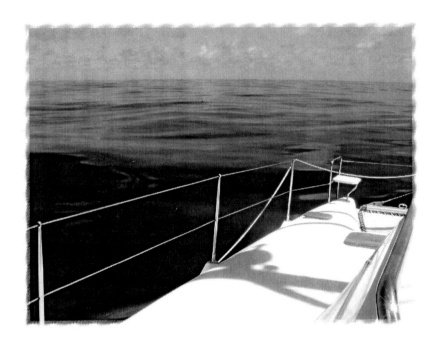

THANK GOODNESS *that after all the hard work of getting to the Galapagos, the islands lived up to the hype. We absolutely loved the time we spent there.*

The first ten days we were totally engrossed in getting the boat back in shape, with the main project being repairs to our plumbing. We were getting tired of losing all of our freshwater on every passage. We made dozens of trips to the small hardware store in town where we became friends with the two young guys who worked there. Between us, we were able to figure out enough words to communicate together, and using what few supplies they had, I was able to jury rig a system that I was reasonably sure would prevent another flood onboard.

A lot of time was spent just hanging around town. In the afternoon we would hit up one of the small restaurants for a very cheap and delicious four-course meal. Then, in the evenings we would head to the main square along the waterfront where the entire town would gather to talk, eat snacks from the street vendors, and watch the men play volleyball.

Unfortunately we were not allowed to cruise the islands freely in our boat. In an effort at conservation, there were strict rules regulating the flow of tourists. The rules actually turned out to be just fine with us. They meant that we got to jump on a tour boat for a few days of pampering instead.

The tour through the islands was amazing. The Galapagos truly are a special place. Ali and I both fell in love with the sea lions who, despite being wild animals, acted more like pet dogs. While snorkeling, they would gather around us, watching intently as we did rolls in the water, and then copied us with spins of their own before stopping to watch us again. They even nibbled at our flippers as we splashed around in the shallow water. It was far and away the most incredible place we had ever been.

JUNE 17, 2004: PACIFIC OCEAN CROSSING
We're underway. This morning I jumped in the water to pull up the back anchor when a sea lion came over and swam with me for a minute. It was a cool way to say goodbye to the Galapagos.

Right now we are slowly sailing along in just six knots of wind. With a month to go, we figure this probably wouldn't be the most prudent time to start using up our diesel. The forecast looks good for the next couple of days, so we will just sit back and wait for the wind to fill in.

JUNE 18, 2004: PACIFIC OCEAN CROSSING
Once again the forecasted winds have let us down. Day one we made a whopping sixty miles, a two and a half knot average. About the speed we would make on a leisurely walk around the park. Three separate times the wind picked up to ten knots and we got up to seven knots with the favorable current. All three times it lasted less than fifteen

minutes. Right now we are motoring again, hoping to get south into the trade winds that are supposed to be around here somewhere.

JUNE 19, 2004: PACIFIC OCEAN CROSSING
The winds arrived last night, and we have been sailing along at a good clip ever since. It feels good to finally be covering a little ground. We're both feeling pretty lazy and tired today. Not sure what our problem is, but we are glad that the boat hasn't required a change in the sails for a couple of days.

I managed to get a little boat work done this morning. Fixed leak number 157. This time it wasn't our freshwater but instead a leaky seal on the raw water pump for the port engine. An easy fix only complicated by the complete inaccessibility of one of the bolts.

JUNE 20, 2004: PACIFIC OCEAN CROSSING
Now we're cooking. Last night we averaged over six knots and today we are doing even better. We should have our best twenty-four hour period ever if this keeps up. Even when we are this far away it is hard to keep ourselves from calculating how long it will take to get there at this speed or that speed. It just doesn't make any sense to do it to ourselves, especially since the good times never seem to last.

The wind and waves have shifted to about 120 degrees off the bow, meaning that they are finally following us instead of having us beat into them. We've been waiting for these conditions for a long time. The boat is incredibly quiet and smooth considering we are sailing at over eight knots.

JUNE 21, 2004: PACIFIC OCEAN CROSSING
Yesterday we logged 164 miles, which is more than our first two days combined. The wind showed up and has continued to howl for over a day now. Fortunately the waves are from behind and only help speed us along while the ride onboard is still very comfortable. We really haven't done anything but lie on the couch and read.

JUNE 22, 2004: PACIFIC OCEAN CROSSING
Great day yesterday. First the fact that we covered 184 miles, which is a record speed for us. Then in the afternoon, still not having any luck fishing, I decided to try out some smaller lures and see if that helped. I threw two different colored three inch squid out and within an hour we had fish on both, a small wahoo and a mahi mahi. Fresh fish sandwiches for dinner.

JUNE 23, 2004: PACIFIC OCEAN CROSSING
Yet another fine day of trade wind sailing. I am finally feeling in the groove of things, in that I don't feel quite so tired anymore; and since the sailing and the motion of the boat have been so good, we have been eating pretty well too. At least a lot better than when the boat is pounding in big seas.

Ali is getting anxious to be there and is not enjoying the thought of two more weeks ahead of us. But she hasn't been feeling all that great either, losing a little lunch over the side yesterday. Hopefully if the sailing stays good she'll start feeling better soon.

Yesterday we hit a new high speed aboard *Bumfuzzle* of 13.4 knots. We were sailing along in beautiful weather when a little rainstorm rolled over us kicking the wind up over thirty knots. We didn't reef, just enjoyed the ride, and it was all over in a few minutes.

Another storm came through a half-hour later. And we thought, boy, we should probably have a reef in and slow things down a little bit. We left the sails alone though, and ten minutes later it passed by harmlessly.

When it looked like a third one was on the way, we finally decided to reef the main and take a couple turns in on the jib. Of course, the next storm never came, and a half-hour later we were shaking out the reefs. I knew reefing was for wimps, the boat was handling the big winds just fine sailing downwind with the waves. Oh well, better safe than sorry, I guess.

JUNE 24, 2004: PACIFIC OCEAN CROSSING

After six full days, we are just over a third of the way there. After a morning lull, the wind picked up again in the afternoon, and by last night we were flying. I woke up at one point and it felt like the boat was going a hundred miles an hour, so I poked my head up to check on Ali and found her sitting at the computer.

"Is everything all right?"

"Fine, no problem," she said.

"It feels like we're flying."

She just shrugged and went back to what she was doing.

Then this morning she admitted that we were actually doing over ten knots when I asked her that. Whatever, once again the boat seemed to be handling everything just fine so I guess we'll take those kinds of speeds.

Yesterday when we were hoisting the main back up, our winch completely died. It hadn't been working correctly for a while now, but the one time I tried to fix it I could not figure out how to get it apart. So when it finally stopped working altogether yesterday, I thought I had better try again. This time I did what most women would have done in the first place, I got out the manual.

I had that thing torn apart in just a couple of minutes, figured out why it wasn't working, and put it all back together without losing any pieces. Then since it was so easy, I tore apart the other one and cleaned and greased it. It's amazing having winches that will actually help when you want to hoist a sail. I probably should have completed that little project months ago.

One other thing that is making this passage so much better than our last is a little addition we made while in the Galapagos. We had a problem with the sink in the kitchen. When they installed it, they ran the drain hose straight down about three feet to a thru-hull drain. Well the problem with that is that when a couple of big waves meet each other under the boat they smash together, and all the pressure from that needs to escape somewhere. Well, it would inevitably escape by blasting up through the sink drain hose, which would then shoot the seawater all over the kitchen.

Even worse was when Ali would be doing dishes and it would blow the drain plug right out and she would have a face full of dirty dishwater. Needless to say, this didn't put her in the best mood. So anyway, the solution we came up with was to add a valve to the hose. So now we can keep it shut all the time, and then when we want to drain the sink we just turn the valve for a second. What a difference that three-dollar piece of plastic has made.

JUNE 26, 2004: PACIFIC OCEAN CROSSING

The perfect sailing weather continues. Today, however, we had to change the sails around. We have been heading southwest with the east wind for the last week but we're starting to get a little too far south, unless we want to tack back north later on. So today we turned the boat straight west and put out the screecher to the port side and the main all the way out on the starboard side, wing-and-wing . Hopefully this way we'll be able to avoid any unnecessary mileage.

JUNE 27, 2004: PACIFIC OCEAN CROSSING

Well we knew things couldn't go on perfectly forever. Yesterday we only covered 140 miles, for our slowest run since day two. The wind has been blowing ten knots since yesterday morning straight out of the east. Running directly downwind for the first time we are realizing it is kind of a pain in the butt. The biggest problem with wing-and-wing is that you need to keep the wind directly behind you. If it shifts too far one way, then the screecher starts flapping wildly, and if it gets too far the other way, behind the main, we'll have an accidental gybe.

Anyway, this morning I woke up and Ali said we needed to switch the sides that the sails were on. We hoped if we did that we would be able to keep the screecher filled better. As we went about doing this we needed to do a controlled gybe and get the main across to the other side. Ali had the line to the traveler in her hands but had unwrapped it from the cleat. As soon as the main gybed the sheet went ripping through her hands leaving her with some nasty rope burns across a couple of fingers. She's okay, just pissed off.

JUNE 28, 2004: PACIFIC OCEAN CROSSING

Yesterday morning, Ali made a nice pancake breakfast for us with the understanding that it was then my job to catch a fish for dinner. Not a problem, we are having a feast tonight. I put out the lines and then laid down for a nap this afternoon only to have Ali wake me up with a, "Fish on!" I ran outside to find we had two huge mahi mahi on each line. We pulled in the first one, knocked him out with a shot of vodka in the gills, and then let the second one go. We're all set for a mighty fine meal.

Last night, we decided to switch the sails around and head farther south, hoping for a more relaxing night watch. When we are sailing wing-and-wing, we have to keep a pretty close eye out for wind shifts and we hoped this change of direction would help that. Once again, though, the screecher wasn't going to allow us to roll it up. We are still completely clueless as to how to roll that sail in if the wind is over ten knots. The top third of the sail will not roll with the rest of the sail and ends up flapping violently and getting all twisted up while the rest of the sail is nicely rolled at the bottom. We quickly gave up and set the sails back out the way they were. We are about ready to unhook that whole sail setup and throw it into the ocean.

Today I was reading a sailing magazine that I have had since Panama. In it there is a page titled Piracy Report. In the short list of places that they warn everybody to steer clear of was good old Buenaventura, Colombia. Yeah, you wouldn't want to go there, that's for sure.

JUNE 30, 2004: PACIFIC OCEAN CROSSING

We have each read half a dozen books since we left the Galapagos. Not simply out of a love for reading, but because recreational opportunities are pretty limited out here. Between reading and playing rummy we're pretty well out of ideas.

The wind has really died down on us. Actually it has just about completely disappeared. We have a thousand miles still to go, and hope this is just temporary.

I was looking at the charts the other day and realized that a straight line from New York to L.A. is only 2600 miles. Imagine putting a car in drive and then idling all that way. That's us.

JULY 1, 2004: PACIFIC OCEAN CROSSING

This sucks. Our nice steady trade winds have abandoned us. We have just eight knots right now and are making very slow progress. The forecast for the next two days doesn't look any better. So what was looking like a very fast passage is starting to look a lot more average.

One thing that has not let up at all is our fishing. We snagged ourselves another big mahi mahi today. Ali and I are having a little debate on who actually gets credit for catching the fish. She puts the lines out in the morning and has been the first to spot that we have a fish on the last three times. Meaning my only job has been to pull them in and beat them senseless with the billy club. Anyway, despite the fact that all our pictures are of me holding them up in the air triumphantly, it's really all Ali's doing.

JULY 2, 2004: PACIFIC OCEAN CROSSING

A very slow day of sailing today, averaging just four knots in very light winds. Beautiful weather if you aren't trying to sail across the Pacific. We had a bird show up this afternoon that seemed to be looking for a place to land, but never did. It's always a surprise to see anything way out here.

JULY 3, 2004: PACIFIC OCEAN CROSSING

Yesterday we were pretty depressed after realizing we were too far away to be able to motor and the forecast was looking bleak, with no wind for a couple of days. Then this morning the wind suddenly went from three knots to fifteen, and after pulling the mainsail up we were rocking along again. Our spirits soared. I sent an e-mail for an updated forecast, and we figured that we were going to find that the trade winds had returned and were ready to carry us the rest of the way.

Then we got the new weather forecast. There are no winds at all predicted for the next three days. Essentially we are looking at being becalmed seven hundred miles from land. Right now the wind is still blowing ten knots and we are managing a pretty good speed. After it's gone I suppose we will be firing the engines up and hoping that they can get us through the next couple of days, after which we will need the wind to return again. It seems amazing that you can be out in the middle of the Pacific Ocean and have no wind and glassy seas.

After that forecast came through, I think we both sank into a mild depression. We are dying to get there at this point.

TODAY I WAS ONCE AGAIN REMINDED how very little I know about boats. I was searching through the West Marine catalog for a winch cleaning and repair kit. As I was reading through it, I realized that it kept referring to one- or two-speed winches. Judging from the description, our winch didn't seem to fit the one-speed category, but the catalog was saying that the two-speed winch should crank in either direction. Counterclockwise at a 1:1 gear ratio, meaning for every turn of the winch handle the drum makes one revolution, and the other direction at a 6:1 ratio.

Intrigued, I went over to the winch and turned it clockwise. Sure enough it spun at a six to one ratio. For eight months I have been raising the main by turning the winch handle six times more than I need to be. What a moron. No wonder I was so exhausted by the time I got the main all the way up.

In my own defense, the winches were both broken before I took them apart, and I am ninety percent sure that the two-speed cycle wasn't working before. Of course all that shows is that I should have fixed them earlier. I'm now really looking forward to the next time I get to crank up the mainsail.

JULY 4, 2004: PACIFIC OCEAN CROSSING

Ali and I were having a good day today. She was busy making all sorts of junk food for us in the kitchen, and best of all, the forecast from yesterday was proving to be wrong. In fact under main and screecher we were making six knots in twelve knots of wind. We were sailing happily along when, "BANG!" We both jumped up and ran outside to find that the screecher was dragging alongside of us in the water.

A second later we realized that the bang was from the screecher halyard exploding. The line snapped right in the middle of the mast, with the top of the line snagging somewhere inside as the sail was flailing about, halfway up to where it should have been.

We quickly dropped the mainsail and began hoisting the screecher sail out of the water and onto the deck. I then heard a really nice ripping noise before noticing that it was snagged on one of the cleats. This produced a foot long tear in the sail. Then we wrapped up as much of the sail as we could with sailties to keep the wind from filling it, which it was doing since the top half of the sail was still up in the air.

Next Ali hauled me up the mast to unhook the sail and secure the remaining halyard. We did that without incident; and half an hour after the bang, we were back underway. Unfortunately we now have to use the jib instead of the screecher, slowing us down a knot in these light winds.

JULY 5, 2004: PACIFIC OCEAN CROSSING

We didn't even bother trying to motorsail today. The wind was non-existent. Instead we spent the entire day running the engines one after another. According to the forecast there is wind on the way just south of us. In an effort to catch it, we altered course and headed in that direction.

It's now five o'clock and we still haven't found any wind. We're really not looking forward to listening to the engines run for another night, but I don't think we have a choice if we want to keep moving. We've only got 450 miles to go at this point. My best guess is that we have enough diesel to motor 300 of that if we need to.

Despite the lack of wind, the weather has been beautiful. Today was ninety degrees and sunny. The water temperature is even warmer than that. In fact it was so hot today that at one point we shut the engines down, and I went for a swim with nothing underneath me for two miles. It's spooky swimming in water that deep, but it is the clearest water I have ever seen, none of the miniature particles of sand and weeds that I am used to. It really felt like I could see down thousands of feet into the beautiful blue abyss.

JULY 6, 2004: PACIFIC OCEAN CROSSING
Man does this suck. It took us just thirteen days to cover the first two thousand miles of this trip, and it looks like it may take another eleven for the last thousand. There is very little wind, with not much more in the forecast.

JULY 8, 2004: PACIFIC OCEAN CROSSING
Wind finally. Not a lot, but enough to get moving and shut down the engines. The wind is coming from directly behind us, so we had to figure out a new way to set up the sails unless we wanted to tack way south and then back north again. We found that we could still sail wing-and-wing without the screecher by running the jib line out to a cleat on the side of the boat instead of through the normal blocks on the top of the cabin. This worked surprisingly well and the boat sailed straight as an arrow.

Only 200 miles to go and we are feeling one hundred percent better now that we are sailing again. We even caught a nice wahoo this morning within five minutes of putting out the line.

JULY 9, 2004: PACIFIC OCEAN CROSSING
It is now the middle of the night, and we're 160 miles from land. As if to play some cruel joke on us, Mother Nature is doing everything she can to keep us from getting there. Yesterday morning the wind started out of the east, by noon it had clocked around to the north, and now it is directly out of the west. Because of the weather today, we now have waves bashing into us from at least three different directions and we have strong winds coming directly from our destination. All this combined is making for some very slow, unpleasant motorsailing. Oh yeah, it is also pouring rain, and a lightning storm has been thrown in for good measure.

We have made almost no forward progress today. Ali pretty much summed up our feeling about it when she said, "There is no fucking way I would ever do this crossing again." After three weeks at sea not a sentence goes by without some potty-mouthed sailor talk splashed in.

JULY 10, 2004: PACIFIC OCEAN CROSSING
After a few more storms throughout the night and early morning, the sea is now almost dead calm again. The sails are down, and we are pointing in the direction we need to go with the engines chugging away.

Our engines each have a thirty gallon tank, and this morning one of them finally started sputtering. We carry twenty gallons of diesel in jerry cans so I dumped five more in each. It looks like we are going to limp in with just a few gallons to spare.

JULY 11, 2004: HIVA OA, MARQUESAS

After twenty-four of the longest days of our lives, we are officially in paradise. We motored all day and night to cover the last hundred miles, and when the sun came up this morning we had the islands in sight.

We motored past rugged sheer cliffs with waterfalls that seemed to spring out of nowhere and shoot down the sides into the ocean below. Dolphins joined us to perform some jumps and added something new we had never seen before. They hoisted their tails high in the air and then slapped them down making a big splash. They stuck with us for an hour and then left as we cruised right through a big group of blue footed boobies that we hadn't expected to see here.

With just a mile to go, the skies opened up and dropped sheets of rain on us, as if to say, you're not getting in that easy. We came around the corner into the bay where we found four other boats tucked in. The guidebook, which is written by a monohuller, said it is a terrible anchorage because it is so rolly. I tell you, I cannot understand why they even bother building monohulls anymore. The monos in the anchorage were swinging back and forth like pendulums while us catamarans sat there nice and steady.

Of course leave it to us to sail 3100 miles only to arrive on a Sunday. We can't check in and therefore can't go ashore until tomorrow. Which is okay I guess, we'll get the boat cleaned up and go to bed early.

Pulling in today was sort of weird, almost anticlimactic. We weren't really excited, just happy to have the hook down again. Maybe it just hasn't settled in yet.

JULY 12, 2004: HIVA OA, MARQUESAS

What was twenty-four days at sea really like? It was boring. Long, tedious, monotonous. Those are the best words I can think of to describe it. Basically, looking back on it, there isn't much to say.

The first two weeks were perfect sailing. We didn't have to do anything. We enjoyed the sun, read a dozen books each, played a whole lot of cards, and thumbed through a big stack of magazines we had been saving since Panama just for this trip. The most exciting times of the day were when we would check e-mail and when we would update the passage log to see how many miles we had covered in the previous twelve hours.

The last ten days of the trip we were plagued with bad weather. Not scary, rough sea type of weather, just crappy weather that we could not sail steadily in. We spent the days making constant sail changes and adjustments, trying to keep sailing at a decent speed and going in the right direction. Meanwhile we kept playing cards and reading. Occasionally the boredom would be broken by dolphins or catching a fish, but that excitement would be over in twenty minutes and then we were back to doing the same thing again. We need a new hobby. Maybe I could knit an afghan.

I think a lot of cruisers won't ever make a crossing like this because of fear. Fear of being at sea for that long. Probably fear of bad weather and rough seas. But based on our experience, there is no reason not to make the trip across other than being bored to death.

With that said though, there is still a very real sense of accomplishment. A sense that we have just completed something that many will dream about, but very few will actually set out and do. However even that feeling is subdued. Maybe that is because this wasn't something we dreamed about for years and years like most people, it is just something that we decided to do one day not too long ago. And maybe that is why we weren't afraid to do it. We just do not comprehend all the danger that is involved. And maybe, just maybe, that's a good thing.

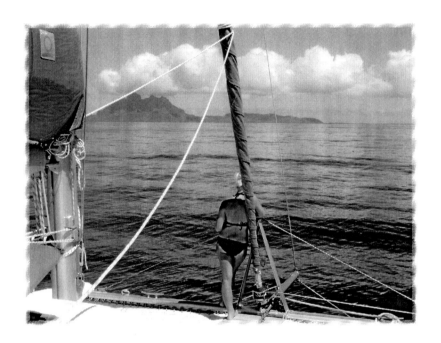

say it people

IT TOOK US A FEW DAYS to actually get cleared into the Marquesas, during which time the rain continued to fall in sheets. To be perfectly honest we were not happy at all in Hiva Oa. Besides the bad weather, we had our dinghy gas tank stolen at the dock, the food prices were astronomical, there were no restaurants, and a beer cost five dollars.

While it was an extremely lush and beautiful place, we didn't find sitting in the dark brown rain soaked bay eating peanut butter sandwiches and papaya to be our idea of paradise. We're all for tropical islands, but after twenty-four days at sea, this was not at all what we had been hoping for. There weren't even any beaches. Now what kind of paradisiacal South Pacific island doesn't come complete with a white sand beach lined with palm trees? After getting cleared in, we were anxious to get moving again and see what the rest of the Marquesas had to offer.

JULY 16, 2004: TAHUATA, MARQUESAS
After a few days relaxing and catching our breath, we raised the anchor and headed for Tahuata just a few miles away. We were only ten minutes outside the bay when a nice squall rolled in out of nowhere.

Squalls have been a pretty common occurrence around here the past few days. This one brought winds of over thirty knots. After a few miles we turned west and rode the wind and waves that the storm produced. We flew along at eight knots with just a little bit of jib out and an engine running to charge the batteries. After two hours we had the anchor down in what the cruising guide calls, "One of the three most beautiful anchorages in Polynesia." And it is beautiful. It has the clearest water we have seen in months, and the beach to go along with it.

JULY 17, 2004: TAHUATA, MARQUESAS
Cruisers are weird, that's all there is to it. Just after the sun came up this morning Ali and I went outside to enjoy it, as it had been at least a week since it had broken through the rain clouds.

As we sat there, we watched the lady on the Swiss boat anchored fifty yards off to the side of us come outside wearing nothing but a t-shirt. That would have been fine I guess, but then she climbed over the lifelines, halfway down the ladder mounted to the side of the boat, squatted, and peed. Now that's class.

JULY 22, 2004: HIVA OA, MARQUESAS
We've run out of propane for our stove and now just have our little four pound grill propane tank remaining. So for tonight's feast we had spaghetti on the grill. We boiled the noodles, warmed up the sauce, and even made garlic bread on it. But better still was last night's dinner of hamburgers and Ramen noodles on the grill. How many

people can claim to have made ramen on the grill? A very select few I'll bet. God, could we use a Taco Bell.

The water here is thirty feet deep, brown, and cloudy, meaning that I can only see what is right in front of me. Today when I went out to check the anchor, I dove down and almost immediately saw a flash of white in front of my face as a huge manta ray swam right at me and then turned up his big white belly at the last second. Visions of being swallowed whole by a shark I never saw flashed before my eyes.

JULY 23, 2004: NUKU HIVA, MARQUESAS
We left Hiva Oa behind yesterday afternoon and sailed overnight to Nuku Hiva, which has a huge bay that juts into the island a mile and a half. It is by far the safest anchorage we have found in the islands and at the head of it is the biggest "city" in the Marquesas.

JULY 26, 2004: NUKU HIVA, MARQUESAS
Ali and I cannot quite figure out what is going on around here. Nobody ever seems to think we are cruisers. The other day at lunner, a cruiser at the table next to us said, "You two must be backpackers, huh?"

Then last night, while at a wedding for a cruising couple, where the only people invited to the wedding were other cruisers, a guy asks us, "So are you two guests at the hotel here?"

We are trying to figure out what makes us so different from the other cruisers. Is it the fact that Ali looks so young, or that I don't have a scraggly beard? Whatever it is, we find it amusing and hope that it continues.

JULY 28, 2004: NUKU HIVA, MARQUESAS
That's it, I can't hold back anymore. The Marquesas suck. The food is terrible, the weather crap, the water dark and murky, and we cannot afford so much as an ice cream cone.

It appears we're not the only people feeling this way either, we met a whole bunch of cruisers last night and everyone felt the same way. The conversation would start out with, "When did you get in?" Followed by, "So what do you think?"

It feels as if everyone is afraid to be the first to mention how disappointing the Marquesas are. The next comment would usually be something along the lines of, "I feel bad for not liking it here, but . . ." Or, "It's beautiful, but . . ."

But it's boring. But it's too expensive. But the food is horrible. But it sure rains a lot. Just go ahead and say it people.

JULY 29, 2004: NUKU HIVA, MARQUESAS
This morning we headed over to Daniel's Bay, which is just around the corner. We got outside the harbor and found the wind howling with gusts near forty knots. Luckily we were only going a couple of miles and it was downwind.

On arrival we found a wonderful bay with 360 degree protection. Once inside we almost couldn't tell where the exit was. We were surrounded by huge cliffs on three sides and a beautiful beach on the other.

Today was hiking day. The guidebook said it was a long and strenuous hike up to Vaipo waterfall, so we grabbed a bottle of water and our flip-flops and headed out. It was a great hike through rainforest and mud. The views and the scenery were amazing.

After about three hours we made it to the waterfall. The cliffs completely encircled us, towering 1000 feet straight up. The waterfall itself was mostly hidden behind a cliff. I went swimming in the pool at the bottom to try to get closer to it but it was like swimming upriver in rapids. It was incredible how much power the falls had. We really enjoyed our afternoon there in a very cool place far from anywhere.

JULY 31, 2004: EN ROUTE TO RANGIROA

We have covered a lot of ground this month, and we are on the move again, headed this time for Rangiroa. We knew the winds were going to be whipping once we got out of the bay and they did not disappoint. Fortunately the direction was perfect as we were headed dead downwind. With gusts as high as forty-two, the highest of our trip so far, we put out half the jib and sailed along very comfortably. Gradually the wind decreased, and we raised the main with a double reef. Yet by late afternoon the wind was down to twelve knots, and by nightfall we were motoring in calm weather.

Today we caught a monster of a wahoo. Ali and I are poetry in motion when we catch a fish. It is like a choreographed routine. I grab the line and keep tension on it while Ali holds the gloves open for me one at a time, like a nurse for a doctor. Then as I pull in the fish, she grabs the hook remover, vodka, billy club, and camera.

I have gotten pretty good at getting the fish aboard and can usually dispatch them without much problem. Pose for a quick picture, and then Ali hands me the filet knife, a cutting board, and a plate to put the filets on. I carve up the fish and hand the plate off to Ali, who takes it inside and cleans it up nice, getting rid of the yucky stuff, and putting the filets in Ziploc bags. Meanwhile I am busy cleaning the cockpit area of fish debris. All of that and we are back to lounging around within fifteen minutes.

AUGUST 1, 2004: EN ROUTE TO RANGIROA

Ali and I have not been able to find our groove on this passage. It's only a five-day trip so we didn't really give it much thought before we left. Then suddenly late on the first day, we both looked at each other and said, God, I do not feel like doing this. Both of us are feeling really tired and lazy, sort of a seasick type feeling.

Luckily the wind has been great and there has been little to do in the way of sail changes. Just set it and forget it. But even the fact that we are going to make it in just four days hasn't done much to change the mood aboard. Hopefully Rangiroa rejuvenates us a little bit.

Now I suppose I should get up and go look around outside since I am supposed to be on watch.

AUGUST 4, 2004: RANGIROA ATOLL, TUAMOTUS

After a great sail in which we covered 600 miles in four days, hardly touching a sail the entire time, we pulled into Rangiroa atoll yesterday morning. On the third day of the passage, we finally came out of our funk, but we were still more than ready to get here.

As we approached the atoll, I had intended to ask for tide information over the VHF. However nobody answered my repeated calls. Our charts didn't have the tide info for Rangiroa, which was a bit of a problem since all the cruising guides stressed that we must only attempt to go through the pass at slack tide. At the wrong time it can be a horrendous entrance.

Not knowing the tides, I was a little nervous about what kind of conditions we would find. Fortunately as we approached the entrance, we saw a large Navy ship go in. I took that as a sign that it must be okay for us to go through also. Maybe not a good idea looking back on it, as I wouldn't imagine that an adverse six knot current would be an issue for a Navy ship.

We pressed on and as we got to the entrance we found some crazy big waves slapping straight up into the air. The current didn't seem to be slowing us down much and it wasn't pushing us along too fast either. Maybe we hit slack tide after all. The pass is about 500 yards long and the whole time we were whooping and hollering as we got tossed around like we were on a wild horse. There were a few small inflatable dive boats full of hotel guests at the edge of the entrance that stopped to watch us, probably thinking that we were completely insane.

Then just like that, it was over. We were sitting atop perfectly calm water despite the twenty knot winds and big seas right outside the pass. That was both the scariest moment and the most fun we have had sailing *Bum* so far.

AUGUST 8, 2004: EN ROUTE TO BORA BORA
The past few days we've really just been taking it easy. We wandered the island a bit, poking around in the shops and visiting the elaborate cemetery. A lot of time was also spent at the hotel bar and swimming pool we were anchored right out front of. That is, until the manager kicked us out of the pool. Rule #4: Pool for hotel guests only.

This morning we raised the anchor and headed for the pass, hoping it would not be quite as wild as coming in the other day. We were relieved to see that it was nearly flat. Maybe having tide information is important after all. The dive shop at the hotel had helped us out with that.

Right now *Bum* is sailing straight downwind wing-and-wing. We are doing pretty well, but with the light winds we are missing our screecher sail more and more.

AUGUST 10, 2004: BORA BORA, SOCIETY ISLANDS
After two solid days of motoring, we arrived in Bora Bora. We had the sails up most of the time, but with winds of only five knots they weren't doing much. I woke up this morning and looked outside to see the island's craggy outline on the horizon, over forty miles away. Being that far away when we spot our destination certainly makes for a long day.

Later in the afternoon, while standing on deck staring at the beautiful island, two humpback whales surfaced just a few hundred yards off the coast. They continued to surface, blowing out a huge spray every time. It sounded as amazing as it looked. We decided to go in for a closer look, slowly motoring in their direction. For a while we didn't see them again. Then suddenly we heard them surface on the other side of the boat just seventy-five yards away. As we continued on toward the island, they slowly disappeared behind us.

AUGUST 12, 2004: BORA BORA, SOCIETY ISLANDS

Yesterday morning we woke to find that there was absolutely no wind. The water was like a sheet of glass. We have not seen water like that since the Bahamas. While out on deck we saw three spotted eagle rays swimming underneath the boat. Another thing we have not seen since the Bahamas.

We jumped in the dinghy and headed out to the nearby reef to find some more. About fifty yards in front of us the water rises from thirty feet to just five. It stays five feet for about half a mile until reaching the outer edge where it comes right up to the surface. That is where the waves from the ocean swell break all day long every day.

We motored as close to the breakers as we could, winding our way through the colorful coral heads and watching as stingrays darted off in every direction. It was an amazing spot with the breaking waves about eight feet high forming perfect tubes in front of us. We sat there awhile admiring the power of the ocean and the beauty of the setting.

AUGUST 13, 2004: BORA BORA, SOCIETY ISLANDS

We seem to have a knack for floods on our boat. Today's came from a toilet thru-hull located below the waterline. It was one of just four thru-hulls on the entire boat that we did not replace in Panama. The fitting was so loose that I could wiggle it with my hand. I tried a few different things to stop the water from literally rushing in, and finally found the answer. A screwdriver jammed into the top edge seems to put it at just the right angle to completely stop the inflow of water. I am really not sure what else we can do while the boat is in the water. I guess we will just sail around for another couple of months with a rusty screwdriver keeping our boat from filling with water and sinking. Nice.

OVER THE NEXT FEW WEEKS Ali and I really got back into the swing of things. After the Marquesas, it seemed every island got better. The weather was incredible day after day. The water was as clear as those we had enjoyed so much in the Bahamas, but filled with even more marine life. Our favorites continued to be the spotted eagle rays which swam around in groups, seemingly in happy little families.

However it seemed the boat was falling apart before our eyes. It felt as if every day we were adding something new to the list of things to fix. That list just grew and grew while we continued to put projects off. It seemed easy enough to just wait on most things since we were heading to New Zealand in just a couple of months. Once there we planned to have the boat hauled and get her back in shape. I knew we would have plenty of time then, so for now nothing seemed all that pressing.

Ali and I were enjoying life on the boat again. The Pacific passage hadn't been hard, but it had taken a toll on us, and we found ourselves not nearly as eager to sail after that. Fortunately the South Pacific weather really cooperated with us, and from the time we sailed away from the Marquesas it seemed the wind just followed us gently wherever we went. We relaxed again. Plus, after a twenty-four day passage, a few days here and there feels like nothing. Skipping between islands was child's play.

AUGUST 25, 2004: TAHA'A, SOCIETY ISLANDS

A year ago today Ali and I were sitting in a mortgage office signing papers on the sale of our condo in Chicago. What a wild year it's been. Looking out the back door right now, at a beach crowded with nothing but palm trees, it is hard to believe. The view here in Taha'a is great, if for no other reason than that there is nobody else around.

SEPTEMBER 6, 2004: TAHITI, SOCIETY ISLANDS

Upon our arrival in Tahiti, there was something that urgently needed to be taken care of. Fast food. When we walked along the boulevard and saw some kids at a playground with McDonald's cups, we knew we were close. As we came around the next corner it appeared, like a mirage in the desert. I'm sure it sounds pathetic, but after cooking for ourselves for months on end, it was great to have old reliable Mickey D's take care of a few meals. And not surprisingly, the locals felt the same way, lining up out the door.

SEPTEMBER 8, 2004: TAHITI, SOCIETY ISLANDS

The cruiser talk continues to center on the robberies along the quay. These morons sit here in the middle of a major city with their boat decks cluttered full of all sorts of good stuff. Then they complain when something goes missing. Ali and I lived in a condo on the ground floor in downtown Chicago, and I assure you we didn't keep our golf clubs and bicycles sitting out on our deck. Yet here in Tahiti that is exactly what the cruisers do.

We spent the last few days checking out the city. We stopped by a couple of marine stores and picked up a few things we needed. We now have the line for our screecher halyard, but have yet to find anybody who can splice the shackle onto it. After three marine stores, a shipping yard, and two yacht charter companies, we have given up. We don't know how to splice a line and it seems nobody else does either. It looks like a simple knot is going to have to do.

SEPTEMBER 10, 2004: TAHITI, SOCIETY ISLANDS

This morning we finally completed our most important boat project, getting the screecher back up. It feels good to have that sail back in the lineup. We have really missed it, even if we do hate it sometimes.

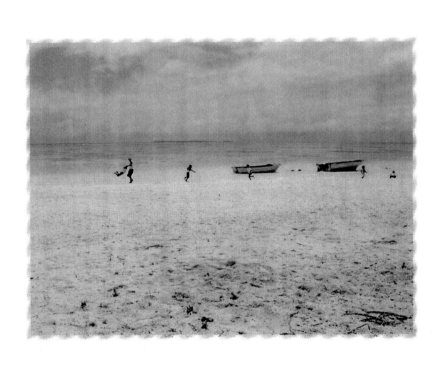

SEPTEMBER 17, 2004: EN ROUTE TO PALMERSTON ATOLL

We spent quite awhile in Tahiti not really doing much, though it felt like we were busy every day. After a few months away, there were a lot of little things to get done, and we needed a major port to find the things to do them. Now with the boat looking and feeling better again, we are ready to take on the rest of the Pacific.

Once we got the boat loaded with food and diesel and ourselves with Big Mac's, it was time to move on. In nice calm weather we motored out through the pass and pointed the bows to the west.

It took until our second night out from Tahiti for any wind to show up, but since then we have had a nice steady fifteen knot breeze. Sailing downwind with the screecher is so easy that it hardly seems worth the effort to raise the main and jib, despite the fact that we could probably make better speed with that set up than with just the screecher alone.

I got seasick yesterday for the first time in months. Not sure what brought that on, but it definitely kept me laid up on the couch all day and night. Ali has been having trouble the last month as well, though she is feeling okay on this passage. It seems weird that we each got a little seasick our first time out in the boat, then were fine for thousands of miles, and now are sick again in relatively calm seas.

SEPTEMBER 19, 2004: EN ROUTE TO PALMERSTON ATOLL

Yesterday the wind slowly diminished, along with our speed. We continued to creep along at three knots while slowly going insane. We are so tired of the food we have onboard that we find ourselves discussing in detail a magazine advertisement with different recipes for macaroni and cheese. "Oh, if we just had some bacon bits and a tomato, or chicken breasts and broccoli. Man would that be the best!" Of course if we did have those things, we still wouldn't want to cook them.

At the moment the wind has completely disappeared and we are motoring. The problem is that with 300 miles to go on this leg of the trip, and 750 miles on the next one, we don't have enough diesel to motor all the way. Soon the engines will have to be shutdown and we will be at the mercy of the fickle winds.

SEPTEMBER 21, 2004: EN ROUTE TO PALMERSTON ATOLL

Under a hundred miles to go now. Yesterday we had been motoring in perfectly flat seas all day, when out of nowhere the wind appeared blowing twenty knots. It will have been eight days at sea when we arrive tomorrow; but aside from our crazy food cravings, neither of us had a hard time with it at all.

We haven't been doing much during the days other than reading and putzing around the boat. I managed to fix a creak that had been annoying me since day one. The wood molding around the doors would rub against the fiberglass whenever the boat flexed, i.e. nearly constantly. It drove me crazy but I could never figure out exactly where it was coming from. Today I finally just started cutting away at the wood until I found the right spot. It is now blissfully quiet onboard. All day I've been talking about how great it is to have the boat quiet at last. Then Ali, sick of hearing about it said, "Well, why the hell didn't you fix it before then?" Point taken.

SEPTEMBER 23, 2004: PALMERSTON ATOLL, COOK ISLANDS

Palmerston Atoll consists of a few tiny islands situated around the edge of a circular coral reef. Only a couple of very small passes lead through the reef to the inner lagoon. Palmerson Island is the only inhabited island, where about fifty descendants of an Englishman named William Marsters still live. Marsters settled the island in 1863, bringing with him two wives and adding a third later. At least some of the family has lived there ever since.

As we approached the island Edward Marsters came out in his skiff to meet us. He showed us where to anchor on the coral shelf outside the atoll, and told us he would be back out at high tide to lead us into the lagoon where there was room for just one shallow draft catamaran.

A few hours later it was time to head in on what would be a nail biter of an entry. The pass was very narrow, leaving only ten feet of safety on either side of us. There were coral heads everywhere, and at one point the depth was just barely four feet. Edward stood up front on the deck, giving me hand signals to steer by, while Ali repeatedly stared over the edge of the boat and then back at the depth finder. All we could do was trust that he knew what he was doing.

He led us through a quarter mile of coral heads and right up to the beach. There he had mooring lines chained onto coral heads ready for us to tie off to. A few adjustments and we were floating perfectly centered between three coral heads, just fifty feet off of a beautiful palm fringed beach in what seemed to us to be about the furthest place on earth from the real world.

We went ashore and walked over to Edward's house where we met his wife and young son David. Edward chopped open a couple of coconuts and David took us on a quick tour of the tiny island before Ali and I made our way back to the boat for our typical post passage twelve hour slumber.

This morning we woke up to find that it was a big day on the island. The supply ship had arrived on one of its three times a year stops. The islanders had placed their orders for food and supplies with family who live on the bigger islands of Rarotonga or Aitutaki. Months later those orders had finally arrived. We spent the morning helping the families transfer their booty from the boat to their homes using wheelbarrows. It was fun seeing how excited everyone was. Like Christmas had come early.

SEPTEMBER 24, 2004: PALMERSTON ATOLL, COOK ISLANDS

Today we went to a funeral. It was for a priest who lived on Palmerston as well as Rarotonga and New Zealand, and whose body had arrived on the supply ship the day before. This is fairly common, as all of the Marsters' descendants consider Palmerston their ancestral home. The funeral service was amazing, held in their small church with walls of windows opening up to views of the beach and the sound of breaking waves.

The hymns they sang were eerie, sounding to our ears like Native American chanting, and led by a very old woman whose voice was haunting and like nothing we had heard before. After the service we all gathered outside the church where the body would be buried. Three men lowered the wooden casket into the grave, fired up the cement mixer, poured it over the casket, and proceeded to quickly fill in the hole. Back home they usually leave that messy business until after the family has left, but here it was all part of the process.

After the funeral the whole island gathered for a picnic. Ali and I were quickly engulfed by all the children and spent the next couple of hours with a dozen kids climbing all over us. It was fun watching the little girls warm up to Ali and ask her to lead them in all sorts of games.

Later on we met another cruising couple who had stopped for the afternoon on their way to Tonga. We were talking about where we had been and where we were going. Apparently they didn't think much of our cruising credentials though, because at one point the lady just looked at us and said, "Oh, you guys aren't real cruisers."

To which we replied, "Thanks, we get that a lot."

Based on the conversation we'd been having, I can only gather that you cannot enjoy big cities and you need to have a love of cooking to be considered a "real" cruiser.

SEPTEMBER 25, 2004: PALMERSTON ATOLL, COOK ISLANDS

The adventures in Palmerston continue. Around noon David started yelling to us from the beach, "Come on, we're going to the birds!"

We didn't have a clue what he was talking about but figured he meant we were having lunch. We asked if we needed to bring anything but he just yelled excitedly, "Come on!"

We headed ashore and walked over to his house where his mother told us they were picking birds. She could tell we still had no clue what everyone was talking about, so she told David to bring us down there to see. We walked down to where we had the picnic the day before, still assuming we were going to some sort of lunch. As we got closer we could here a strange noise. It sounded like pigs squealing. A pig roast for lunch? Then we saw it. All the islanders were gathered around a net with dozens of squawking birds in it; little fuzzy Boson birds.

Every month, from June to October, a few men go to a nearby *motu* to collect the birds. They leave the momma birds behind and collect their babies, who are six weeks old and too young to fly. A total of six hundred birds are picked each year.

This month there were forty-three birds. I'm not sure how they divide them up, but Edward had a clipboard and told each family how many they would get. When he gave the word, all of the kids that were gathered around the net jumped in and started grabbing the crying birds, throwing them into their respective families wheelbarrows. The kids thought it was great fun, while we just stood around stunned by the whole scene.

Afterwards we went back to Edward's house. The entire family was already hard at work preparing the birds for the next day's feast. I figured that if I was going to eat any Boson birds I'd better help out, so I grabbed one of the squawking birds, gave his neck a good snap, and started picking feathers.

Once the birds were picked clean one of the children would take a machete and chop off the wings. They then handed them to mom who would shove a stick in them and hold them over the fire to singe off any remaining feathers. Next the bird was sent over to grandma who was in charge of gutting them.

One of the kids told me I was lucky they didn't get more birds today, usually they get around a hundred and it can take until dark to finish all the work. Ali, fortunate not to have been given a Boson bird assignment, kept busy with a few of the little girls that are hanging off of her at all times.

We are definitely getting the full experience of life on Palmerston. Ali and I were joking that we will have spent more time in church here in one week than we have in our entire lives.

SEPTEMBER 26, 2004: PALMERSTON ATOLL, COOK ISLANDS

This morning we woke up and went to church. Our souls are now saved, and from what I could gather we will indeed be going to heaven. Before church we went to Edward's where we found everyone lying around in their shorts, showing no intention of going anywhere. They told us David had just left and that they would see us afterwards. So we walked off on our own.

The service was surprisingly short, and afterwards everyone gathered outside. All the old ladies came up and welcomed us once again. Each taking their turn approaching us for kisses on their cheeks. They are the sweetest ladies and it is fun to see how they are treated in this society. Here everyone respects their elders without question. If grandma says jump, they jump.

Back at Edward's, after a quick rehashing of the day's verse and a recital of the Lord's Prayer, everybody sat down for the baby Boson bird feast. I cut Ali and I a nice clean piece of breast meat while the rest of them cleaned every ounce of meat off the bones. Edward told me the best part of the bird was the fat attached to the skin and then proceeded to watch me closely. With no other choice I grabbed a chunk of fatty skin and bit into it. Mmmmm, gulp, yummy.

After lunch we had a few of the kids out to the boat for a swim. They had more fun than I would have ever thought possible just jumping off the back of the boat into the water over and over again.

At three it was off to Uncle Bill's Yacht Club for ice cream. Now there was a treat we wouldn't have expected on an island that only has power for a few hours each day. Bill is a super nice guy who asked us to spread the word that he is a full-service yacht club. What that means is that he can fix an outboard engine, he has the only clothes washer on the island, and he will offer you every single item of food that he has. All he asks in return is that you bring him some cheap Panamanian beer.

SEPTEMBER 27, 2004: PALMERSTON ATOLL, COOK ISLANDS

Palmerston is not an easy place to leave. Everybody on the island has welcomed us with open arms, asking nothing in return for their hospitality. It's strange to think that we'll leave here tomorrow with very little chance of ever returning. But that is just the way it goes on this tiny atoll in the middle of the Pacific.

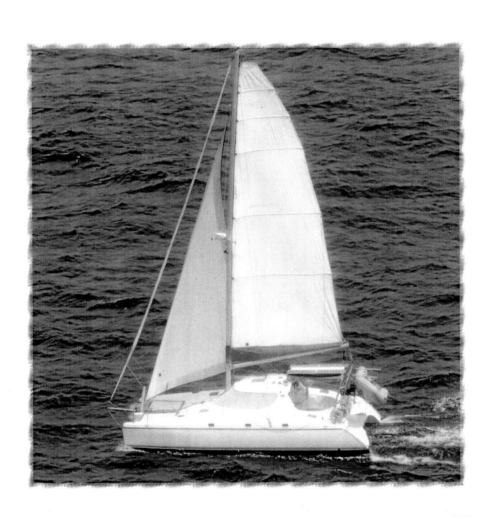

a lot to learn

SEPTEMBER 29, 2004: EN ROUTE TO TONGA

A couple days ago we bid a fond farewell to all of our new friends in Palmerston. At high tide we ran the gauntlet out of the lagoon without any mishaps and were soon on our way to Tonga.

By night the wind had picked up enough for us to enjoy a nice sail under a full moon so bright that at times it looked as if a ship was shining a spotlight on us. Since then the wind has been behind us at around ten knots and we continue to make slow but steady progress.

A funny thing happened the day before we left Palmerston. Another yacht had arrived and we were sitting around shooting the breeze with them at Edward's house. While talking about how some cruiser was having trouble anchoring outside of Palmerston the lady said, "I tell you, some people think that you can just hop on a boat and go. Well I don't think so, there's a lot to learn." Ali and I just looked at each other and rolled our eyes.

Then the conversation shifted to Tahiti and we mentioned how happy we were to eat at McDonald's after all those weeks at sea. They both gasped and said, "We *never* eat fast food, but you're American, so . . ." Maybe they didn't see the Tahitian cars lined up around the block to go through the drive-thru. After that enlightening conversation Ali and I politely excused ourselves.

After our last couple of conversations with the yachties crowd it has become clear that we have no business being out here in the same waters as them. It feels to us like we need to conform to what the narrow-minded vision of cruising is supposed to be, or at least pretend to, in order to fit in.

OCTOBER 1, 2004: EN ROUTE TO TONGA

As has been the case for most of the South Pacific, this has been a pretty slow passage. We have a major crack in our bimini support, which we are worried enough about that we have decided not to use our mainsail until we can have it welded. With so much relying on that frame, we don't think it's worth the risk. Fortunately the screecher has been the only sail worth using so far anyway.

We caught a couple of nice mahi mahi on this trip. No matter how many lures I buy the only one that works is my old generic pink and blue squid that is half missing from being chomped off. The hook is so rusted it looks like it could fall off at any minute, but the fish still love it.

OCTOBER 2, 2004: EN ROUTE TO TONGA

We had a pretty exciting encounter today when a false killer whale decided to join us. I was lying on the couch staring out the back door when I saw a huge fin float past us. We both jumped up and ran outside where we found a whale, about twenty feet long, swimming right alongside of us. He swam at the surface lazily and then drifted underneath the boat. He stayed like that for a few minutes before making a slow descent and disappearing.

The island of Tongatapu was well situated both as a rest stop and a jumping off point for New Zealand. We spent a few days there recharging ourselves after a string of 500 plus mile passages across the South Pacific.

After making a couple of essential repairs, we set sail again. It was an exciting time, knowing that this was going to be our last sail for a few months. We were ready to settle down in a place for more than a few days or weeks. It amazed us just how exhausting life on a boat could be at times, and the prospect of not moving for a while held great promise for us.

OCTOBER 15, 2004: EN ROUTE TO NEW ZEALAND

It is day three of our sail to New Zealand, and I can finally write a log. We enjoyed our time in Nuku'alofa, Tonga, most of which was spent just hanging out in town. It's an interesting place, ruled by a beloved King, who's seemingly torn between their traditions and western civilization. Many of the men wore wraparound skirts, called a tupenu, with what looks like a handwoven straw mat over that. The shops sold a lot of intricately woven handicrafts right next door to the internet cafés and pizza parlors. It was a great town to just sit and people watch, as it had a little of everything.

The reason I couldn't write the last few days is that the wind was just off the nose and the boat was really bouncing. I have never been so seasick. I could not keep anything down, not even a sip of water. But when I woke up today I was perfect. Ali wasn't feeling it too bad. She was smart enough to take a Dramamine before we even left the harbor. She probably wished she were sick though, so she wouldn't have had to listen to me moaning and complaining the whole time.

Last night on the charts there was a tiny speck listed only as a rock. It said the depth was unknown and I figured it was just a submerged rock, but we altered course to pass a good six miles away from it anyway. At four a.m. I looked over and could see a mountain, even in the dark. As the sun came up two hours later we saw a huge island, at least a mile long. I wonder how many boats have run smack dab into that thing in the middle of the night. It is on a direct line between Tonga and New Zealand. After that, we started giving everything a wide berth. Reefs that were marked with a depth of 130 feet, didn't matter, we steered well away from them.

OCTOBER 18, 2004: EN ROUTE TO NEW ZEALAND

The winds have been light the last three days, and we have been either sailing slowly or motorsailing. We have around 450 miles to go. Another five days out here during which time the winds are forecast to spin around on our nose.

In Tonga, the boat next to us hired a weather routing service to figure out the best route to follow on this passage, and he offered to share it with us. We gladly accepted, though now I am having nightmares about it since we usually don't pay much attention to weather and have always been fine. So far it has not shown us anything that we didn't already know. In fact they seem to be an exact copy of the free e-mail weather file that we have been using since leaving Florida.

Some cruisers spend hours every day gathering weather data. I always found it to be a little overkill and was especially amused by it in the Bahamas. Why, when you are only a couple miles from a safe anchorage at any given time, would you spend your entire morning listening to weather forecasts, downloading weather faxes, and who knows what else? We would hear people talking about it every single day and could never understand it.

I don't have a clue about weather forecasting, and yet by downloading this one simple e-mail every few days I know as much as the guy who spends hours with headphones on trying to listen to a weather forecast over the radio from 2000 miles away, or even a company that specializes in weather routing. But still, every cruising book drones on and on about how to read weather faxes, and what it means when a high pressure system moves over a low pressure system, when the pressure is dropping, blah blah blah blah. Seems like a waste of time these days.

OCTOBER 20, 2004: EN ROUTE TO NEW ZEALAND

Holy crap is it cold. The temps have been falling steadily since we left Palmerston a few weeks back. Now it is just getting unbearable for us tropical babies. This morning Ali admitted to me that last night she even turned on the oven to warm it up in here.

The passage continues to suck. The wind has been consistently out of the south, right where we need to go. Fortunately they have been very light winds.

OCTOBER 21, 2004: EN ROUTE TO NEW ZEALAND

Finally, a break in the monotony. We just got buzzed by the New Zealand Air Force. He had to do two fly-bys since we didn't have our VHF on. Ooops. He wanted our names, boat information, as well as where we intend to land. So I guess the Kiwis should be all ready for us when we get there now.

OCTOBER 23, 2004: OPUA, NEW ZEALAND

After a much longer than we had hoped for passage, we arrived in Opua around noon. Clearing in was a simple process. We've got almost no food on the boat at this point, so about the only thing the quarantine officer could find to take away from us was the dirt in our vacuum cleaner. Now we're just looking forward to five months of passage-free living.

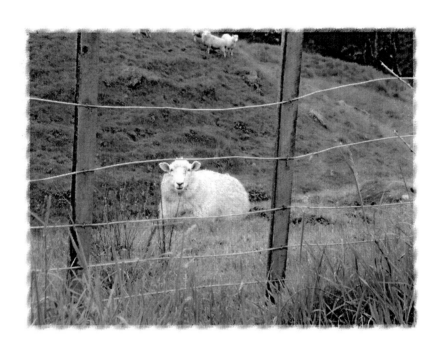

NEW ZEALAND WAS TREATED as a time for us to regroup. The past year had been a huge adjustment for us; and though I felt that we had done incredibly well, I knew that this break couldn't have come at a better time. At this point sailing hadn't really grown on us. We thought of the boat simply as a mode of transportation, a place for us to sleep at night. It was clear that Ali had no love for sailing, but she'd never wavered in her determination to continue on with what we were doing.

The part of cruising that we really enjoyed was experiencing the different cultures. Usually when somebody says this, they follow it up with some lame story about visiting a village on a tour bus and having the natives do a dance for them. And let's face it, the route we had traveled through the South Pacific, aside from Palmerston Atoll, was heavily touristed. Those were the types of cultural experiences most were having.

We gave up on the idea of South Pacific savages early on, realizing that for the most part the people weren't much different than us. For us, experiencing a culture became more about joining people in going about everyday life.

This is one of the real benefits to the cruising lifestyle. It wasn't just flying in and out for a week, never leaving the hotel. With cruising, we were forced to do the same things the locals did every day. Shop for groceries at the stores or in the markets, get fuel, track down spares at the hardware store, use the internet cafés, and visit the post office.

Our days were absolutely consumed with these simple, mundane chores. But our absolute favorite travel experience was merely sitting down at a restaurant with a cold beer and a view of the street to watch the world go by.

New Zealand was the perfect place for us to do all of those things. We slipped easily into the life of an expat. With Bum on the hard for a couple months worth of delamination repairs we were always eager to get away. We bought an old Volvo for fifteen hundred dollars and began crisscrossing the island. Soon there wasn't a road left on the North Island that we hadn't highlighted in our road atlas.

At Christmas we made our first, and only, trip home. It was exciting, and we were eager to share our experiences with our friends and family. Within just a few days, reality set in though. Nobody really cared about what we were doing. That sounds too harsh. They cared, but it just wasn't reality to them. It had been over a year since we had been home, but it felt like it had only been one day. Nothing had changed. Life had gone on without us just like it always had. Everybody still had work, commutes, bills, kids, and snow to shovel off the driveway. We had very little in common anymore and it showed. By the time we got on the plane back to New Zealand we were ready, and excited to continue with our travels.

JANUARY 27, 2005: WHANGAPARAOA, NEW ZEALAND

After nearly three months, we are getting ready to put *Bum* back in the water. Today we had the riggers out to reinstall the mast. While working on the wiring one of them asked Ali for the Windex. So obedient Ali, thinking he wanted to clean the mast, went and grabbed him the bottle of Windex and a roll of paper towels. The look on his face as Ali handed him the glass cleaner was priceless.

He held it for a few seconds before bursting out laughing. Turns out he wanted an entirely different Windex, a twirling piece of plastic that goes on top of the mast to show the wind direction. A wind indicator I guess. We had always just used the one on the cockpit controls that showed a boat and an arrow. Who wants to look straight up at the top of the mast anyway?

FEBRUARY 8, 2005: WHANGAPARAOA, NEW ZEALAND

Today I was painting our rusty barbeque propane tank. I had this cool spray paint that leaves things feeling rubbery. Well it turns out the paint was nearly the same gray color as the fabric on the boat, and since I was having so much fun with it I asked Ali if I could spray the man overboard pole too, more commonly referred to as the flag pole on our boat. The MOB pole was painted dark red, which didn't match at all, although I am guessing there may have been a safety issue involved there. Now it is this sweet looking gray that really ties in nicely with our color scheme. A classy choice indeed.

WITH THE MAJOR BOAT REPAIRS wrapped up, we loaded into the Volvo for one more road trip. We drove to the South Island where we spent a month marveling at the majesty of the snowcapped mountains and the rolling green hills. New Zealand is easily one of the most beautiful places on earth. It's also one of the most fun.

The South Island is adventure central. We jet boated along glacial rivers, bungy jumped from one of the highest and most dramatic settings in the world, and sledged down class IV rapids with nothing but a wetsuit and a small plastic sled.

Bruised and full of adrenaline, we returned to Bum, sold our car for one hundred dollars less than we paid for it, and prepared to leave.

MARCH 16, 2005: WHANGAPARAOA, NEW ZEALAND

We are almost ready to go sailing again, and honestly we are pretty anxious to get to it. It has been about five months since the boat left the marina, the longest time in one area that we expect to spend on this trip. It's strange to be feeling a little nervous about sailing again. Actually not the sailing part so much as just going to sleep with the boat tugging at an anchor instead of tied up to a dock.

The small boat projects are getting done now, and our four page list has just about every item crossed off. We were wondering today if maybe we should have left a few things on the list to do when we are back on the water. As it is now, we shouldn't have anything to do but relax once we get back out there.

Ali has three ducks that come by the boat at least three times a day. They'll stay for hours, waiting patiently for more bread while Ali holds a conversation with them. I'd swear they are talking back to her too.

Yesterday I was working on the front of the boat and when I walked to the back I found one standing on the dinghy straining his neck for a look inside to see if

Ali was coming out with his lunch. When he saw me he just quacked and looked at me like, where's the lady with my lunch?

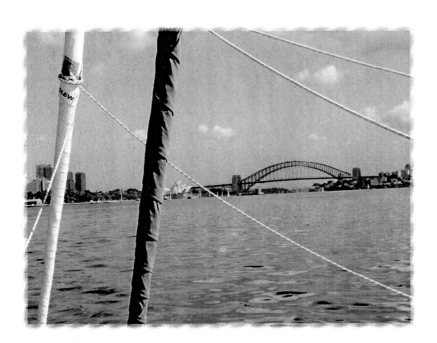

APRIL 21, 2005: TASMAN CROSSING

While clearing out with customs yesterday, we received a stern warning that we must leave immediately and not stop anywhere along the coast. We were to go directly from Opua to Sydney. That seemed a little excessive to us. We didn't see what had suddenly changed that made us such bad people that we could no longer be trusted to step foot on New Zealand soil. Yet because of this I can't go into any detail as to how we spent the night.

I got up early this morning to check e-mail one more time before heading out. The weather still looked good, and after a couple more hours of sleep we were on our way.

We headed out with winds on the nose, then tacked further east and motorsailed for most of the morning until the wind picked up. Just as forecasted, a storm blew past us from the south causing the wind to shift, allowing us to cut the motors.

For a couple of hours we were knocked around a bit. Ali had just started to make lunner and I was sitting at the helm, when the wind died down to eight knots, a very noticeable change causing Ali to come out and say, "What is this, the calm before the storm?" About a minute later the boat veered violently into the wind which had jumped to thirty-five knots.

We had full main and jib out and were seriously overpowered. The wind had hit so hard and fast that we hadn't even a second's notice to prepare for it. I turned off the autopilot, took the wheel, and was able to get us back on track, but the wind was still howling. Ali got the lines ready and we raced around putting a double reef in the main. The whole time Ali was repeating, like a mantra, "We're gonna die, we're gonna die." It cracks me up every time she says that because we always live through it. Then just as quickly as it all started, it quit. The wind dropped down to twenty and we were once again sailing comfortably.

After that less than stellar start, we sat down and had a little pow wow to hash out some ground rules for the passage.

Rule #1: when somebody says the words "calm before the storm" we shall immediately double reef the main.

Rule #2: we would reef the minute the wind hit eighteen knots and double reef at twenty-three knots. Amazingly, the boat seems to sail just as fast, but we feel much more in control.

Rule #3:   we would sail with one reef in at night and would put the
second one in at twenty knots.

Rule #4:   we would actually follow rules one through three.

APRIL 23, 2005: TASMAN CROSSING

Day two of the Tasman was great. We continued to have moderate winds on the beam
all day and covered a lot of ground. We are finding ourselves to be a little overcautious
so far, reefing early and often, but have decided to sacrifice some miles in order to not
get caught with too much sail out. We've been extremely careful at night, sailing with
the first reef in even with winds at only fifteen knots. It is probably silly, but the peace
of mind is worth it, especially at night when we can't see the weather that is
approaching us.

Today started out with the wind dying and shifting to the southwest, causing
us to head north a bit and off our direct line to Sydney. We motorsailed for a few
hours before the wind picked up, and we were able to cut the engines and get back on
course.

Now we are enjoying a beautiful day. The sun is shining, the waves are small,
and *Bum* is making five knots. We cannot ask for much more than that while crossing
one of the most feared seas in the world.

We seem to have licked our seasickness problem. For the first two days out,
we took a couple of Dramamine pills. The effects have been great. We have never felt
this good so early into a passage before.

APRIL 25, 2005: TASMAN CROSSING

I think all the people who have said that we have just been lucky with the weather so
far are going to have to start giving us a little more credit. Here we are five days into the
Tasman and we have had nothing but perfect sailing weather. At the moment we have
a nice following breeze and are surfing down the waves at seven knots. Perfect.

Last night things got a bit breezy with winds at thirty knots. It was from the
side so not a big deal, though we did get pooped pretty good. The waves had built up
quickly and didn't have a lot of space between them. The boat would lift up on a wave
then slide down the back side before immediately being picked up by the next one.

Every once in awhile the second wave would hit before one side of the boat
had a chance to make it down the first wave, leaving us slanted right into the oncoming
wave. One finally broke right over the boat as Ali was sleeping and I was on watch. We
always have the cockpit doors open, so all I could do was watch the wave wash into the
cockpit, ricochet off of the seats and flow right in through the doors. There's nothing
like a little late night flood clean-up.

Other than that, things have been pretty uneventful. It has basically been a
normal trade wind passage, which is exactly what the Tasman Sea is not supposed to be.

APRIL 27, 2005: TASMAN CROSSING

It seems the Tasman has had a change of heart. Yesterday morning the wind suddenly
kicked up and spun around on our nose. It wasn't predicted to be anywhere near there,
and yet there it was.

We spent hours tacking back and forth, making little progress as the waves continued to build throughout the day and night. Thankfully this morning they died down to virtually nothing, and we were able to get back on course and start putting some miles under the keels again, though this time with the engines.

When we received our weather forecast today, it warned that we have got a nasty front coming from Sydney in about 48 hours. Bringing big winds, the likes of which we have never had to deal with before. They are predicting thirty knots, with squalls over fifty a virtual certainty. Then over the course of a day, the wind should shift from up ahead of us to back behind us again. The timing couldn't be any worse, as by then we will be only two hundred miles from Sydney.

Other than that bit of news there hasn't been anything of interest going on out here. No fish caught, no dolphins or whales spotted, nothing other than a few albatross and other assorted sea birds checking us out. Sometimes it seems all we do is sail and read. Sail and read.

APRIL 29, 2005: TASMAN CROSSING

Only 250 miles to go now. Yesterday was the most perfect day; perfect to be lying on a beach. It was hot, not a cloud in the sky, and not a breath of wind. Not exactly ideal for trying to race towards landfall in a sailboat.

After twenty-four hours of steady motoring the wind finally filled in last night, allowing us to sail. Unfortunately we're still expecting that nasty weather front to show up soon, which is going to make for a pretty uncomfortable ride.

Ali is a bit nervous over what we are going to do if the fifty knot winds do show up. Options include heaving-to, as well as just running downwind for a few hours while the weather works its way around us. The only thing she really wanted to hear from me though, was that we weren't going to try to bash head on through it. Once I promised her we would find a way to take it easy on ourselves, she felt a lot better.

At this point we are extremely excited to get there and are really hoping for only two more nights at sea. We have both been in high spirits on this passage, which I think is because we were both secretly dreading this trip. Well maybe Ali wasn't so secret about it. The truth is that the Tasman's reputation for bad weather and rough seas is something you just can't ignore. But because those haven't shown up, life onboard has actually been really nice.

APRIL 30, 2005: TASMAN CROSSING

Now we're just plain desperate. It is five p.m. and we have exactly ninety-eight miles to go. We are running both engines at the moment, something we never do, because we want to get there so badly. The passage hasn't been bad, but my original worst case scenario of ten days expires tomorrow morning; and if we don't make it in by then, I am afraid Ali isn't going to believe me the next time I tell her how long a passage will take.

I said ten thinking more realistically that we would make it in eight or nine and everybody would be happy, but a couple of days with wind on the nose screwed up that little plan. Again though, we can't complain, we seem to have made it across the Tasman Sea without a scratch.

Yesterday's big winds did show up, but not quite as strongly as we had feared. In the morning the wind quickly picked up to thirty knots, where it stayed the entire day. The sky was clear, which was nice, since we didn't have any of the squalls we had been warned about. The waves built throughout the afternoon, Ali guessed fifteen feet, and I said twelve, though honestly neither of us has any idea how to make an accurate estimation of wave height. What we do know is that they took us on some pretty wild spins, making for a long wet day.

Amazingly, right before dark the wind died down. It never does that. Instead it always seems to get worse, so that we have to spend those hours that we can't see anything wondering what is about to hit us. We were pleasantly surprised and enjoyed a nice sail all night, until this morning when the wind completely disappeared and we had to fire up the engines again.

A little after midnight, we experienced a big lightning storm, which was a first for us. It is truly amazing to watch one of these storms out at sea. It is something we give no thought to while living on land, but out here, when we know our boat is the only thing for hundreds of miles sticking up fifty feet in the air, it can be a little unnerving. We unhooked as many electronics as we could and settled in to watch the show. The vertical lightning was striking in a 180 degree arc in front of us but thankfully managed to always keep a few miles away. The horizontal lightning would light up way off to the south and reach in a spider web all the way over our heads. We were happy that the show never got any closer.

MAY 2, 2005: SYDNEY, AUSTRALIA

The past couple of days were tough on us. Two nights ago promised to be our last night of the passage. We were motoring along in variable winds, for the most part light and on the nose. Not a big deal as we had enough diesel, and if we just kept plugging along we would be in Sydney by noon.

Then at two a.m., with only thirty miles to go, the wind began to pick up quickly. An hour later it was holding steady at over thirty knots and was coming directly out of Sydney to our west. The forecast hadn't said anything about this, so initially we thought it might not last long. We raised some sail and headed northwest.

Eight hours later the wind had not let up and we were suddenly closing in on land, now thirty miles north of Sydney. We kept thinking that if we could get into the lee of the land, the wind and waves wouldn't be so bad. But then as we got farther and farther north, the wind began clocking around to the south, the direction we now needed to go. We were so close now, but couldn't seem to get any closer.

We got to land around noon and began tacking back out to sea. I was pretty sure at this point that we wouldn't have enough diesel to get us down to Sydney, but after an hour of sailing back out to sea we decided to screw it and just pound south and see when we ran out. I kept two gallons in a jerry jug just in case. We were motoring slowly because of the waves, and it was beginning to look like we wouldn't make it in before 10:30 p.m. which is when customs went home for the night.

Eventually we caught a small break as the wind shifted just enough to allow us to motorsail and pick up our speed a bit. Finally, at nine o'clock we steered the boat through the Heads and into Sydney Harbour. We grabbed a customs mooring, got cleared in, and went to bed. The Tasman Sea had been conquered.

THE NEXT MORNING we slipped away from the mooring early. The Sydney Opera House and Harbour Bridge were just a mile farther on and we were anxious to sail past them. I think for any sailor, steering your own boat through this historic and beautiful harbor is a terrific accomplishment. For me it ranked up there with transiting the Panama Canal. It wasn't so much the act of what we were doing as it was the setting in which we were doing it. A few locations would sum up our circumnavigation, and this would be one of them.

Available dockage is scarce in Sydney. Inexpensive dockage is doubly so. Ali and I somehow managed both. After inquiring at half a dozen marinas, we were beginning to resign ourselves to the fact that we were going to have to settle in quite a few miles from the city center. Then we spotted a young guy on a dock out front of a small field of moorings. He seemed to be in charge so we motored towards him and Ali yelled out, "Have you got any open moorings?"

The kid looked up at us through squinting eyes and asked, "You Yanks?"

"Yanks? I don't know. Pat, are we Yanks?" I nodded in the affirmative. "Yep, Yanks."

He paused a minute, eyeing us up, and said, "Yeah, I suppose I could put you up."

We were thrilled. We'd scored a mooring in about the most prime location in downtown Sydney. It was only eleven o'clock but it was time to celebrate our arrival. After tying up we went ashore. It turned out the kid on the dock, Chris, was also the marina manager. He was more than happy to flip over an Out to Lunch sign and join us for a few beers.

We stayed a month in Sydney and fell in love with the place. We made a lot of friends, including for the first time, website friends. Sometimes it seems that there are more boats than people in Oz, and a lot of them had found our website, followed us along, and invited us out. One guy took us up in his airplane and let me fly, another took us out to a Rugby match, another on a downtown Sydney pub crawl, and a few more out to dinner. It was overwhelming, but would continue from one end of Australia to the other. We didn't stop without meeting up with somebody new.

When it came time to settle up our tab for the mooring, Chris was happy to accept an old anchor we weren't using as payment. A few nights earlier a group of us had been detained by the Australian Navy when we made a drunken three a.m. dinghy trip through a restricted area in order to reach a favorite late-night hot dog stand. We escaped any serious trouble by letting our Aussie friends blame it on us Yanks. So maybe accepting such a ridiculous payment was simply repaying us for that. Either way it was a great ending to an exceptionally fun stop on our trip.

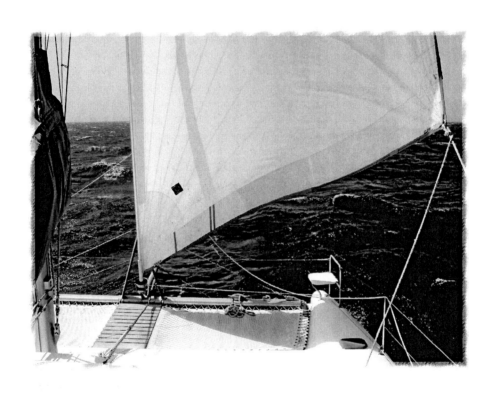

we hesitated

JUNE 1, 2005: NEW SOUTH WALES COAST, AUSTRALIA

It was surprisingly hard to leave Sydney. We were tied to a nice safe mooring a quick walk away from anything we could possibly want, on the doorstep of an incredible city. But when we woke up the other morning and found the temperature inside the boat was fifty degrees, we knew it was time to start heading towards the equator again.

After a few weeks off, we kept our first day of sailing pretty modest. It was extremely modest in fact, only motoring an hour to the other side of the harbor. Today, however, we ventured back out to sea. A huge swell was running into the harbor; but once we got around the headland and pointed north, it gave us a nice push.

We had the perfect wind for the screecher sail and were somewhat amazed when we shut off the engines and simply sailed up the coast in peace and quiet. What a novel idea, using just the sails to propel the boat in a forward motion. After an uneventful morning we rounded the corner into Pittwater. We headed straight for a little bay full of empty moorings surrounded by a national park. Then for the first time in a month, we just stayed on the boat and relaxed.

JUNE 4, 2005: PITTWATER, AUSTRALIA

We met a cruising couple today who have never ventured offshore, but who think they might like to. Their one recurring question revolved around what the long passages are like. I should really consult a thesaurus, because the only word I can ever seem to come up with is boring.

We spend hours and hours for days on end with nothing to do. The boat doesn't require our constant attention. Between the sails, engines, and autopilot, it's got things pretty well covered. Of course there are a lot of exciting moments out at sea like, catching a big fish, having dolphins join us, spotting whales and finding water in the bilges. Then there are always a few frantic moments when the wind picks up or quickly shifts and we are required to take action. But for the most part there just isn't a lot to do. We are sailing the trade wind route around the world for a reason.

We each reach a point on every passage when we say, this sucks. And at the time we say it, we really think it does. But once we make landfall all is forgotten, and we are two of the happiest people in the world. I always feel a real sense of accomplishment at those moments. Ali never used to think much about the achievement of sailing across vast oceans, but yesterday when we were talking to this couple she seemed genuinely proud when she said, "Yeah, we crossed the Tasman." I think she may have even had a bit of a swagger about it.

JUNE 9, 2005: LAKE MACQUARIE, AUSTRALIA

Today we anchored right in the middle of a sailboat race course without realizing it. Dozens of boats sailed past us while Ali and I kicked back in the sun with a couple beers and watched these guys (guy to gal ratio of 100:1) race around in circles. Actually race seems like a strong word for what they were doing. They were moving at under two miles an hour. Can that really be called racing? No matter how hard I try, I just can't see how that could be fun.

JUNE 19, 2005: NEW SOUTH WALES COAST, AUSTRALIA

The weather has been awful the last couple of weeks. The trade winds this time of year are supposed to be from the southeast, which would be absolutely perfect for sailing north up the coast. Unfortunately we have not gotten those winds. Instead we have had nothing but winds from the north or the west, forcing us to sit tight on the northerlies and run for the next stop on the westerlies.

The most recent forecast showed a one-day window with winds from the west sandwiched between a few days from the north. So we decided to leave Coff's Harbor at one a.m. yesterday for the sixty-mile trip to the Clarence River. We motorsailed in light winds through the night until the wind picked up in the afternoon and we were able to cut the engines.

We arrived at the Clarence River entrance by two o'clock and prepared for our second river bar entrance. The trick with these river bars is the tides. During a flood tide, the water from the ocean floods into the river creating a current that runs upriver. This leaves a relatively flat sea at the entrance. During an ebb tide, however, the river and the ocean swells collide, making the area very messy and rough. We didn't know at the time just how big a deal this could be.

ABOUT A WEEK AGO we entered our first bar entrance at Lake Macquarie. The day was similar to yesterday with light winds of five to ten knots and a small swell. When we got to the entrance, despite it being an ebb tide, the water was like glass and we were able to continue right in.

Yesterday, at the Clarence River entrance, I expected to have similar conditions. Again, there hadn't been much wind for the last couple of days and what little wind there was came from the west, which seemed to be mellowing out the swell. So despite it being near the end of the ebb tide, I figured that we would see similar conditions to Lake Macquarie.

The cruising guide told us there were breaking waves about a quarter mile out from the entrance and that to avoid these we should sneak in close to the end of the breakwall before entering the runway. The runway is an area about a hundred yards long that runs between two long breakwalls directing the river out in to the ocean.

As we approached the entrance, neither of us noticed anything out of the ordinary. There were a few waves breaking against the north wall, but that made sense because of the small south swell. Then just as we entered the runway, we saw a huge wave about seventy-five yards in front of us that seemed to be moving in slow motion as it rolled straight up the river. Looking back now it would have been at this point that we probably had five seconds to make the decision to stop and get ourselves out of there. But we didn't, we hesitated, and then it was too late.

Suddenly there were huge breaking waves roaring up behind us. Ali scrambled to close the cockpit doors while I tried to get the boat pointed in a straight line up the river. The waves were on us in seconds. The first one picked the boat up what felt like a hundred feet in the air, but somehow passed safely underneath us. We weren't so lucky on the next one.

The wave took control as it grabbed hold of the boat. Up to this point I had been using the autopilot; but I realized now that wasn't going to react fast enough, so I hit the standby button and grabbed hold of the wheel. I cannot imagine how fast the boat was moving at this point. For the moment we were pointed straight ahead and I still had hope that this wave too, would slide beneath us. If not, the fear was that we could be pitchpoled. Essentially we would do a somersault.

Then suddenly the boat veered to the right. We were in the face of a huge wave, sideways at a forty-five degree angle, and moving at incredible speeds. We could see the wave beginning to break and we were completely under its control. It seemed at that moment there was no possibility of a good outcome. The boat, with us on it, was about to be flipped over and smashed against the shallow river bottom. The wave continued to break from one end to the other, until the top of the curling green monster above us finally turned white and crashed over the top of our heads.

Ali was knocked off her feet and slammed to the cockpit floor by the wall of water, while I somehow managed to hang onto the wheel. It was in the split second as the wave broke over us that we both truly thought that it might be all over for us. It was hard to imagine how this was not going to hurt. We had zero control and were completely at the mercy of the wave as it passed both over and through us.

Miraculously, the boat didn't flip. Then, despite the fact that we were still moving sideways at an unbelievable speed, I was able to crank the wheel and feel the boat slowly come back around.

There were more waves gathering up right behind us though. I yelled to Ali to stay in the cockpit, hammered the throttles and kept going, trying desperately to keep the boat running perpendicular to the oncoming waves. The cockpit was full of water as the drains couldn't keep up, and the doors had popped open a crack when the wave hit, so there was a lot of water inside as well, but so far no serious damage. We held our breath as a couple more waves lifted us up, passing harmlessly underneath before breaking violently upriver. And then, just like that, we were out of it.

The whole thing happened so fast that we could hardly believe it had happened at all. We motored into calm water, both shaking, not sure if it was because we were wet and cold or because our nerves were fried. I suppose it had more to do with the adrenaline coursing through our bodies. We both stripped out of our soaked clothes and Ali brought up some dry ones to put on. Ali kept asking over and over again if I was alright. I just sat there in stunned silence.

Ali went inside to make sure the bilge pumps were doing their job and that everything else was okay. Somehow the computer was still sitting on the nav station table charting our progress as if nothing had happened. A half-hour later we were tied up to a mooring where we spent the rest of the day cleaning the boat in silence.

Aside from learning a lesson on how severe these river bars could be, we also learned just how seaworthy our boat was. There is a lot of criticism directed towards catamarans by monohull owners, but I have no doubt this same situation would have ended very differently if we had not been on a cat. I was also assured by the fact that by keeping our heads we can make it through pretty much anything. Neither one of us panicked, which enabled us to get things under control and get out of there in one piece.

THIS INCIDENT, no matter how much we may not have wanted it to, changed things for us. Before it happened we were completely fearless. Invincible. Afterwards, we were different. Ali became very nervous in following seas. We had always loved running downwind with the waves rolling up behind us. But now, even what would have previously been considered just an average size wave, was cause for concern. As for me, I really felt like I had let us both down. This was something that could have easily been avoided; but because I hadn't, we now had lost some of our carefree attitude.

JUNE 24, 2005: NEW SOUTH WALES COAST, AUSTRALIA
We waited nearly a week before we moved again, but as the wind had finally shifted it was time to go. We motored into the river, confident that we had the tide figured out and that there wouldn't be any waves. Yet as we entered the swiftly flowing water we were sure we could see big waves forming a mile away at the entrance.

Ali called the Coast Guard on the VHF and they assured us that now was the time to go. We motored hesitantly forward and found there were no waves, just calm seas welcoming us back out. The waves we thought we had seen were nothing more than the swell against the horizon.

Sailing up the coast that afternoon I was sitting outside reading a book when a pod of about fifty dolphins appeared at the front of the boat. They all took turns swimming in the bow wake for a few seconds but then within a minute they were gone. I didn't see them surface again anywhere.

Seconds later my attention was drawn to the side of the boat by a flock of squawking birds, diving at the water. Usually that meant fish were being chased to the surface. As I looked over, a humpback whale suddenly breached twenty yards from the boat. His giant head broke the surface first, before he slowly arched his back, gave a big guttural groan, lifted his tail, and dove. He was so close I could see clearly the color and texture of his skin.

I jumped up and yelled to Ali, scaring the crap out of her in the process. We could still see the area where the whale had just dove, leaving a turbulent oil slick behind. We held on tight as we waited for him to surface again, but he didn't. Just like the dolphins, it seemed he had just come up to have a quick look at us before going about his business.

JUNE 27, 2005: NEW SOUTH WALES COAST, AUSTRALIA
It never really dawned on us before, but a lot of people, upon hearing the name of our boat, assume the meaning has a much more European influence. We Americans don't often use the word bum. Yet overseas the name *Bumfuzzle* seems to make women blush and hesitant to repeat it.

Today we got the best reaction yet when the wife of the mechanic working on our engine asked for our boat name?

"*Bumfuzzle.*"

"Excuse me?"

"*Bumfuzzle*," we said again.

When she realized she had heard us correctly she gave us an angry look and actually used the words, "Tisk, tisk." We quickly explained the meaning to her but still just got an unhappy shake of the head.

JULY 10, 2005: QUEENSLAND COAST, AUSTRALIA

Sometimes it seems the coast of Australia is nothing more than a series of river bar crossings. After motoring overnight we arrived this morning at the Wide Bay entrance. This bar has a pretty notorious reputation around these parts. In fact just a few weeks ago, it flipped over a forty-two foot catamaran, so we were paying extra attention on this one.

As the sun came up we found that we were just one of about ten boats heading for the bar. We filed through one after the other, a couple of boats even leaving a sail up.

The bar has one section called the Mad Mile; and even though we were going through at the perfect time and with very little swell, we still got a sense of how ugly an area it could be. Fortunately we motored right through without problem, and after a few more hours up the Great Sandy Straits we dropped the anchor.

We hadn't been settled for more than fifteen minutes when a customs boat pulled up alongside of us. They asked for our cruising permit, and then asked who named the boat. I blamed that on Ali while she was inside getting the paperwork. Everything seemed to be in order, so they took off, and we took a nap.

JULY 16, 2005: QUEENSLAND COAST, AUSTRALIA

We spent the last couple of days hanging out at Lady Musgrave Island. The wind was over twenty-five knots out of the north for two solid days, and when it calmed for a few hours on the third day, we raced the dinghy ashore. The island was all coral, which is always a little strange. It sounds and feels like we are walking across a beach full of our mother's best china with large chunks of coral clanking against each other.

Other than that little outing, it was just too rough to bother doing much of anything. We pretty much stayed cooped up in the boat other than a couple of quick dips in the water to check the anchor and make sure we weren't moving around. Sometimes this lifestyle can seem awfully monotonous. The bad weather we have had since leaving Sydney is really starting to wear on us.

This morning we left on a two-day sail up the coast. The forecast for the next four days called for south winds around fifteen knots and that is exactly what we had this morning when we left. But somehow a few hours later we once again find ourselves motoring into a north wind. It's only about five knots and I'm sure it won't last, but for some reason this seems to happen on every trip lately.

JULY 20, 2005: QUEENSLAND COAST, AUSTRALIA

When I left off, we were motoring into the wind on our way to Percy Island. A couple of hours later the wind did shift back to the southeast and we had a nice sail. Actually too nice because we made such good time that we arrived at Percy Island at two a.m.

With very little wind and not very detailed charts, we decided to just drop the sails and float a couple of miles out from the anchorage until morning. We probably could have gone in using the radar, but it just didn't seem worth it. This is the one thing that Ali thinks I may be overcautious about. I really hate to make a night approach anywhere, no matter how obvious and straightforward it looks. As the sun came up, we motored in and dropped the anchor just out from the beach.

One thing I am having a hard time getting a handle on along the Australian coast are the tides and currents. The tides are huge. Right now they are about fifteen feet from high to low, and these create strong currents of at least a couple of knots, even well out at sea. I mention that because this anchorage, in addition to strong winds and a crappy swell, also has a nice strong current running through it. It took everything I had just to swim against the current fifty yards to check on the anchor.

We went ashore in the afternoon and found a beautiful beach. The sand was so fine that as we walked across it our feet made a squeaking sound. Like when we were kids and would drag our tennis shoe clad feet in the hallways at school. When it first happened we both stopped and said, "Did you hear that?"

That night I got an updated forecast and it was looking ugly, with twenty-five knots plus for the next few days. So first thing in the morning we decided to make a run for it. Airlie Beach was about 130 miles away, and we should have been able to get there by early the next morning, before the worst of the weather.

As soon as we got out of the lee of the island the wind kicked in. We were racing directly downwind flying only the jib, which I tied off to a cleat on the side of the boat to help keep it filled. The seas built throughout the day and by noon they towered over us. They were well spaced and coming from directly behind so we rode them pretty comfortably, but it seems that after our bar crossing experience the nerves might not be what they used to be.

We received another updated forecast, now predicting gale-force winds. At about the same time, a squall came through kicking the winds up over thirty-five knots. Between our shot nerves and the weather forecasts, all signs were now pointing to the closest exit, which was Mackay Marina twenty miles away. With the wind shifting around to the east it would remain a straight downwind ride. The problem with this plan was that we wouldn't make it to the marina before dark and would have to enter at night. On the plus side was the fact that this harbor is the world's largest sugar loading terminal, and was sure to be well lit.

We continued flying downwind with the wind now at forty knots and the seas huge, but consistent. A couple of hours after dark we made the approach to the harbor. As we expected, it was glowing brightly. We rolled through the entrance without a problem and headed towards the marina.

The waves were smashing against the outside breakwall and the spray was washing over it in sheets. When we got into the marina area I dropped the engines into neutral and tried to call the marina office to get directions on where to go. As soon as I put the engines in neutral we began washing towards the dock. I put the engines in reverse but quickly realized that reverse wasn't going to be strong enough to stop us and instead jammed them into full forward, spinning away from the docks just in time. The wind was so strong that even behind this huge breakwall we were being blown around like a toy.

Our VHF calls were eventually answered by a few boats in the marina. The office was closed, but they told us to come around the pier and they would come out to give us a hand with the lines. Within minutes the rain began to come down, turning the ugly weather into simply nasty conditions. I circled around while Ali got fenders out and lines ready. By the time we got to the dock, we found half a dozen people standing out in the wind and rain ready to help us. It was really nice of them, because with the weather like it was I don't think there is any way we could have gotten in safely without them. We were tied up securely within five minutes and everybody went home cold and wet.

The boat was yanking so hard on the dock that we had to double up all of the lines in order to give us some peace of mind. This morning as I type this, the wind has not let up and the rain is coming down sideways. Needless to say, we are happy to be in here and not out at sea.

ALI MADE THE COMMENT at one point yesterday, "I didn't think sailing up the coast of Australia was going to be so much work." Me either. From everything I had read I was expecting a leisurely sail up the coast with friendly southeast trade winds blowing us gently along in short little day hops from secure anchorage to secure anchorage. Instead what we have had so far are north winds and southeast gales. It's been a much more challenging coast than I would have ever expected. Thank goodness we've been having such a good time whenever we aren't sailing.

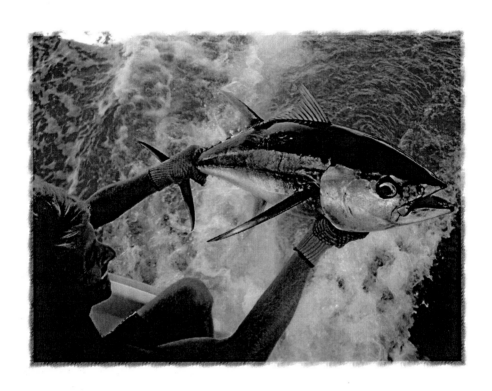

JULY 26, 2005: WHITSUNDAY ISLANDS, AUSTRALIA

In the never ending search for the source of miscellaneous water leaks around the boat, we removed a ceiling panel today and found one in the fiberglass base of our compass. I wish they hadn't even installed a compass, we've never used the thing and now we find a leak because of it. Anyway, after a little epoxy and a fresh caulk job, we've got another leak checked off the list.

Ali is busy at the moment doing the dishes. A job that she hates one day and doesn't mind the next, but which nevertheless needs to be done. She experimented with letting the dishes pile up for a couple of days between washings but then found that she always hated to do them because it took so long, so now she is back into the daily routine. My job that I can't stand doing all the time is lowering and raising the dinghy. It's just such a hassle. My ideal boat would have a davit system that would allow me to leave the outboard motor on permanently.

That got me thinking about how much our roles on the boat are like a couple from the 1950s. Ali does all the cooking and cleaning, while I do all of the manual labor. It's sort of strange because our lives in Chicago were so gender neutral. We ate out every day, so no cooking and dishes. We lived in a condo, so no mowing the lawn. We both walked to work and barely ever drove anywhere, so I didn't even have to do that. Now that I think about it, I really didn't have to do anything back home.

Something else we have realized this past year is that cruisers are the nosiest people on earth. After a quick swim today, I rinsed and toweled off on the back of the boat. As I was doing this I could clearly see the guy in the boat nearest to us staring at me through binoculars, and even me staring back at him didn't persuade him to stop.

I'm not sure, but I think people on boats believe that binoculars have a super power that makes them invisible as long as they are held to their eyes. It sure seems that way. For the record, they are not invisible. I know because we see them all the time. I mean come on, you never find your neighbor on your nice suburban street sitting in his living room window staring across the street at you with binoculars. Or at least if you did you would call the police. I don't know what makes it okay to do it on a boat. It's creepy.

AUGUST 20, 2005: NORTH QUEENSLAND COAST, AUSTRALIA

Every night the cruisers in this anchorage get together on the beach for drinks. We knew this within five minutes of our arrival because two dinghies came by to tell us. I was slightly disturbed by one man's use of the phrase, "cocktails and nibblies," quite sure that I'd never heard a man use the word nibblies before. But whatever, last night we went ashore to meet everybody.

Ali and I are always a little wary of these get-togethers. They tend to go like this: polite introductions all around, a few words about what design our boat is, and then somebody invariably asks how old we are. This is followed by a few hearty chuckles and at least half the people telling us they have kids older than us. At this point the conversation fades into an awkward silence and we begin to feel like party crashers at a geriatrics convention. Fortunately last night, at the point where they tell us they have kids our age, two of those kids stepped forward and introduced themselves. They were a couple who were sailing with their parents for a few days, and we were able to sit and have a nice conversation with them without feeling like complete oddballs for a change.

One issue that came up in conversation last night, that we can never quite understand, is this whole buddy boating thing. Cruisers just love to buddy boat, sailing from place to place in the company of other boats. I understand wanting to travel with friends and enjoy new places together, but I don't understand why everybody has to leave at the same time and sail as close to each other as possible. Why can't they just meet up once they get there?

One lady's face lit up after hearing that we were heading to Darwin. She said, "Oh, you have to talk to so-and-so, they're going to Darwin as well. They're leaving tomorrow and the two of you can sail together. How nice."

We smiled and nodded and thought to ourselves, why in the world would we want to sail with this other couple that we have never met, and suddenly be forced into making all of our decisions as a group with them?

We can sort of understand it when sailing in scary pirate infested areas where you feel that security blanket will somehow make you safer. But even then we don't really get the concept. Wouldn't a pirate's eyes just light up if he saw a group of four unarmed boats instead of just one? Unless one of the boats we are sailing with is carrying a machine gun onboard, what could they possibly do to help us in a pirate situation? I don't know, I guess we'll leave that subject alone until we actually get to one of these areas and have to decide if we want to sail as part of a group or not. I'm leaning towards not.

AUGUST 22, 2005: NORTH QUEENSLAND COAST, AUSTRALIA

This afternoon I finally rigged up a replacement lure for the good old pink and blue squid, our favorite lure that disappeared recently. This one is an exact replica of the old one, except that it still has all of its skirt and doesn't yet have the rusty hook and leader.

After rigging it up I gave it a squirt of WD40 and dropped it in the water. Within a few minutes we had our first bite, a small tuna. We released him and threw the line back in. Ten minutes later we caught and released another small tuna. Then five minutes later we had another fish on. This time when I grabbed the line to pull it in, the 250# test line wasn't budging. This fish was fighting hard. After a good ten minute struggle I had him right behind the boat but still had no clue what it was, as he had yet to surface.

After twenty minutes I finally lugged him up onto the back step and saw that we had yet another tuna. Only this one was a huge yellow fin tuna, around thirty pounds. The beauty of tuna is that once you have them on the boat they completely stop moving. It's as if they are afraid if they move you will see them. Kind of like the cruisers with binoculars.

This guy just sat there stiff with fear while I unhooked him, held him up for a picture and threw him back in. I can hear the gasps from the sushi lovers around the world, but with Ali talking to the fish the whole time telling him it was going to be okay, there was really nothing else that I could do.

SEPTEMBER 6, 2005: GULF OF CARPENTARIA, AUSTRALIA

We are three hours from Darwin and the end of our Australian sailing. We didn't get much wind for this last sail and motored nearly the entire way. There are some strong currents running along this track, and we found ourselves motoring at only two knots at one point but as much as eight at others. It didn't seem to strictly coincide with the tides either, so we never knew what we were going to get.

In addition to the tides there is a thick brown algae in the water. It's pretty nasty stuff and plays tricks on our eyes, making it seem like we are sailing into a coral patch. We wouldn't want to run the watermaker here, but otherwise it seems pretty harmless.

We are extremely excited to get to Darwin at this point. We think we might have bitten off a bit much by deciding to sail to Sydney and cover the entire east coast of Australia in just three months. We covered nearly 2900 miles, which is equal to sailing from New York to Miami and then south through the Caribbean Islands not stopping until South America. It wouldn't be so bad if we were just sailing the distance in one shot, but when trying to fit in as many other things as we were, it was exhausting.

While this is not quite the mid-point of our trip, I still thought some of our statistics were interesting. So far we have sailed 14,500 miles. Ali and I have sailed overnight 108 times. That's 216 three-hour shifts, or about 3000 miles each at an average of five knots. Miles that we have sailed by ourselves while the other person slept. We have been gone a little under two years, around 600 days, meaning roughly one night out of six has been spent on an overnight passage. Not to mention the countless day hops, of which there were at least a hundred.

Here are some other fun numbers. We have used 645 gallons of diesel fuel at an average cost of $3.09 USD per gallon, just under $2000, or roughly $100 per month. I can only estimate, but I would say that one quarter of that was used at anchor to charge the batteries. Another quarter was used to motorsail, which on average adds about two knots to our sailing speed. The remaining half we used for straight motoring, which by using only one engine at a time at relatively low RPMs gives us a speed of 4.5 knots. Fuel consumption is also close to half a gallon per hour.

So what does all that mean? If correct, it would mean that we have motored/motorsailed about 3500 miles out of those 14,500 and that every mile motored cost us 56 cents. Of course, other than the amount of fuel and the cost, the rest of those numbers are just guesses, but I think they sound about right.

SEPTEMBER 13, 2005: DARWIN, AUSTRALIA

When we returned home the other night we found a business card from customs stuck on our boat. Handwritten on the card was, Call me ASAP. That can't be good. We called them the next morning, and as soon as I said there was a note left on my boat she said, "Ohhhhh, you must be *Bumfuzzle*." Again, that can't be good. Her tone was friendly though as she went on to explain why they had been looking for us.

Turns out our cruising permit had expired on August 1st, the same time our original visas had been set to expire. We'd had our visas extended but completely forgot about the cruising permit. She went on to explain that customs hadn't heard from us since we checked into Sydney. That wasn't entirely true, we had spoken to customs a couple of times along the coast when they had approached us at anchor. But I wasn't going to mention that because according to their rules we were supposed to contact them at every new port. Obviously we had never done that.

Now with our cruising permit expired, and nothing showing that we had checked out of the country, they were wondering where we were. Then the day before, she had been wandering through the marina when she just happened to notice *Bum* sitting there.

Fortunately she was very friendly and didn't seem all that concerned about any of this. She just politely asked us to come down to their office with our permit and get the extension.

I decided to press our luck and explained that we were on our way out the door for a trip down to Uluru. Could we do it when we got back? She just laughed and said that she would make a note in the system about when we were planning on clearing out of the country and told us to have a great trip inland. Nice. I love government officials that don't take themselves too seriously.

SEPTEMBER 25, 2005: DARWIN, AUSTRALIA

With the days ticking away, Ali and I have been forced to once again dive into boat projects. Yesterday our work day was cut short by something much more important though, the footy final between the West Coast Eagles and the Sydney Swans.

I've become a big fan of "the footy", as the Aussies call their Australian rules rugby. Ali is always up for watching the games as long as she doesn't have to pay attention to it, and can just sit and enjoy a beer. So at noon we found ourselves back in the familiar surroundings of the Lizard Bar and Grill downtown, a place we have been spending far too much time at lately.

During the game we met a group of guys who work as independent cameramen and sound crew for the news, documentaries, or whatever. One of them is shooting a show for National Geographic and asked us if we wanted to be in it. About the only thing we know at this point is that there will be some night swimming involved. The other day at the croc park the ranger told us, "To swim at night in the Top End is suicide." So that sounds fun.

SEPTEMBER 28, 2005: NATIONAL GEOGRAPHIC ON LOCATION, AUSTRALIA

The other night when we returned to the boat, a guy from National Geographic approached us and said he and his colleagues were sitting at the marina restaurant and would like to invite us over for a drink. We had been playing phone tag with the production assistant all day, and were relieved to hear she was at the restaurant as well, so we could get the details for tomorrow.

As it turns out they were actually staking us out, and after a little chat told Ali that they were considering her for the main character, a German girl who was in Australia on holiday when she got snatched by a saltwater crocodile. Sweet! Well, not sweet that a girl got eaten by a croc, but sweet that Ali got to play her. Then they told me that one guy would have a bigger part than the others, and that I looked liked him so that would be my part. Alright!

After they told us we had the parts, we broke the news to them that we didn't own any hiking gear. No shoes, no shirts with big pockets all over them, none of it. No problem they said, they would take us shopping.

YESTERDAY MORNING WE ARRIVED at the hotel early and were whisked away to the outdoor outfitters in Darwin. They quickly had us trying on shoes, shirts, and hats. They bought us what we needed and then we headed over to the hotel to pick up the rest of the actors. The other actors were a group of backpackers from all over the globe, not an Aussie in the bunch. Then we were loaded up into a big truck, all nine of us, for the hot drive to Litchfield National Park. Ali and I had driven the exact same road a week earlier so it wasn't all that exciting to see Litchfield again.

When we got to the location for the first shoot, we changed into our hiking outfits in the wardrobe department. The wardrobe department consisted of wrapping a big beach towel around our bodies while we shimmied in and out of our clothes underneath. Fortunately for them we're not jaded actors just yet.

All changed into our hiking gear, they then began wiping dirt all over Ali, spraying her with water and generally trying to make her look like she had been out in the bush for a couple of days. Nobody else was receiving any attention and it quickly became clear to everybody who the star of the show was.

Before long Ali was yelling, "Cut! Cut! I can't work in these conditions! Where is my Evian water?!" Things like that. The rest of us lowly extras were getting resentful, and I was trying desperately to disassociate myself from her. The film crew seemed to love her though. They had her doing all sorts of cute little flips with her hair and fake giggles, which she pulled off perfectly. Every scene was set up around, where should Ali be for this shot.

It was great fun and I was super proud of her, but I couldn't show that in front of the girl extras or they would turn on me and call me a traitor. We extras have to stick together.

Next up was a daytime swimming scene which went pretty well and was a nice cool-down from the heat. After that we loaded up and moved locations to the camp scene where we all sat around the fire after a long day of hiking, played the didgeridoo, and generally acted as if we were having the time of our lives.

They spent some time with everyone doing close-up shots, but once again Ali was queen, and they spent hours shooting close-ups of her face and getting as many thoughtful/excited/sorrowful/happy/confused looks as they could get out of her. About this time some of the other girls started asking the director if their characters even had names. He quickly made some up and the girls scampered off happily reciting them.

A little before midnight we wrapped for the day. We found out that tomorrow's shoot wouldn't start until six p.m. so Ali and I decided to catch a ride back into Darwin instead of staying with the other actors in the local motel. They all took off and we watched the cameramen setting up the lighting for the climactic nighttime swimming scene.

The spot was beautiful and the water crystal clear. The park ranger was on hand and assured us that there were no crocs in this area, not even freshies. That helped put our minds at ease and we are really looking forward to the shoot tomorrow. CUT!!!

SEPTEMBER 29, 2005: DARWIN, AUSTRALIA
"National Geographic presents, the beautiful, talented, and famous, Alison Foxx in her inspirational debut on the American television screen. Also starring Sir Patrick Schulte, International Man of Mystery."

Ali's agent decided that she needed to change her name to sound more sexy and less German. I don't have an agent and just thought Sir Patrick sounded cool. I was wrong, and should definitely get an agent.

What a day yesterday. The crew picked us up and we drove back down to Berry Springs, the location of the night shoot. Along the way we stopped to pick up a take-out menu from the restaurant that we would be ordering from later. In the parking lot of this roadhouse bar restaurant we noticed a sign out front advertising, TOPLESS Barmaid 5:30-7:30. Since it was only 5:15 we just stayed in the car while one of the crew ran in.

I wasn't sure a strip joint along the highway was a good sign of things to come, but in the end they served a pretty good beef and black bean on white rice. Yes, we broke every rule ever written about eating at strip joints, even rule #2, don't eat Asian food. Rule #1 of course being never eat anything at a strip joint.

SETTING UP FOR THE BIG SCENE was really cool. The swimming hole we were using looked spooky at night. As they were getting the lighting in place, hundreds of fruit bats circled and dipped into the surface of the water. It was creepy. Fortunately the bats left as quickly as they had come, but not before one of them first left a squirt on Ali's head. She turned and went on a screaming tirade at her assistant for not holding the umbrella over her head properly. Or she would have, had she been that type of bitchy actress. Or had she had an assistant, or an agent, or really anybody to yell at.

The night shoot went really well. We still had to do take after take of the different shots, but the director seemed pleased with the results. It was funny though, we were all swimming about the same amount of time, but the girls were able to tread water much longer than the guys. I was exhausted and could hardly move my arms by the end. Same for the other guys, we were all panting and would fight over the small rock that we could stand on for a few seconds of rest. Meanwhile the girls happily floated on their backs or casually paddled around in circles. Meanwhile us guys would sink like bricks the second we stopped our furious kicking and paddling.

Ali was the big star of the show and the night shoot definitely made that clear. It was really awesome how great she did. Her big scene, getting yanked underwater by the croc, gave all of us the chills. Seriously, it was wicked stuff. The director immediately said that it would be the clip that would play right before every commercial to keep the audience coming back.

I had a pretty major part as well, and may even end up with a dramatic yelling scene, assuming it doesn't land on the cutting room floor. At three a.m. we finally shot the last scene, and after an attempt at snapping a group photo in the pitch black darkness of the woods, we were on our way home. The whole experience was great and we had fun with it.

Nice side benefit to this little television adventure is that it paid pretty decent as well. At least it covered the damage I did to our rental car last week. We can never get ahead lately, but scratching our way back to even for a couple of days is nice.

WE RECEIVED OUR CAIT and social letter for Indonesia yesterday. The CAIT is the cruising permit that we need in order to sail in Indonesian waters, and the social letter is needed in order to stay more than thirty days. With the paperwork in hand, we went to the Indonesian embassy in order to get our visas. The embassy was right downtown and the paperwork was straightforward and easy to fill out. The only problem is that it takes four business days to complete. So it now looks like we will be here until next Thursday instead of Tuesday.

After that stop it was time to visit Australian customs to fill out more paperwork and set up an appointment to be checked out of the country. Our customs officer was training a new guy, which we have found makes things go more smoothly somehow. He didn't even yell at us about that expired cruising permit of ours.

We have been watching the weather to Bali and it doesn't look like we will be sailing much. We bought three more jerry cans that fit in our chain locker, which brings our total to ninety gallons. That should give us enough to motor pretty much the entire way if needed.

OCTOBER 3, 2005: DARWIN, AUSTRALIA

We just heard the news that there have been terrorist bombings in Bali once again. It's hard to fathom that there are people in the world who would purposely target innocent civilians, but it seems it is an inescapable truth these days. From the sound of things on the news, Australians are flocking home in droves. We're not interested in changing our plans based on terrorist actions though, so we'll be on our way to Bali in a few days.

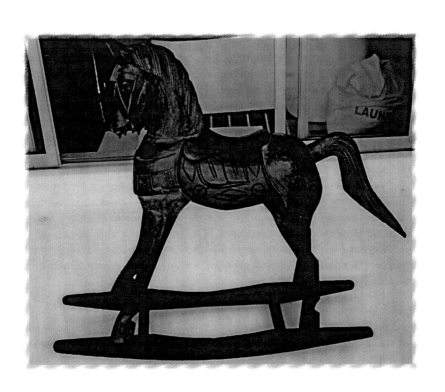

have fun in Bali

There was this weird guy hanging around the dock the other day who fancied himself a Jesus wannabe. He wore greasy hair, a stringy beard, and a rice sack like a toga. While I was tying up the boat, he walked over and asked me what the blue things were on the side of the boat.

"Those are fenders."

"Oh cool. So they're like weights to keep the boat from tipping over?"

After looking him in the eye and determining that he was dead serious I said, "Yep, without them we'd be sunk."

At six we fired up the engines and were on our way. As we pulled out of the marina the sun was setting and was right in our eyes. There were two markers outside the marina, one a red buoy which we were supposed to stay next to, and the other a yellow marker which marked a dangerous shallow area.

We couldn't see very well, and couldn't make out any colors at all; so after frantically discussing it, we headed for the larger of the two markers. One marker was just a tiny little thing floating in the water looking like it hardly belonged there, and the other one was a large buoy. I guess it should have made sense that the dangerous area would be marked with a larger buoy; but it didn't, and we ended up with a very close call. We just skirted alongside the yellow marker and saw the depth climb all the way up to six feet. The eighteen foot tides saved our butts there. An hour earlier and our fenders would have been the only thing keeping us afloat.

After that less than stellar start we were on our way to Bali. The forecasts had continued to show little to no wind, so we were a bit surprised when we actually had fifteen knots on the nose for a good portion of the night. Thankfully by morning the wind died like it was supposed to, and we dropped the sail and put up the bimini side awnings for some added shade.

Around midnight I woke up to Ali screaming. I jumped out of bed and ran upstairs to find her standing in the doorway looking at a two-foot-long fish flapping about wildly in the cockpit. He had flown right past her head as she stood outside having a look around. I'm not saying Ali orchestrated the incident, but the timing was suspiciously convenient as she then got to go to bed fifteen minutes early.

Now sitting here in the middle of the afternoon, Ali rolled her head towards me and mumbled, "It's hot." In fact, it is damn hot out here. Even the water temperature is ninety-six degrees, the same as the air. On top of that we are running the engines to add that extra bit of heat. It wouldn't be bad if only we were sitting on the beach enjoying a cold beer and a swim. Yikes, day one, and we are already talking like that.

OCTOBER 8, 2005: EN ROUTE TO ASHMORE REEF

Three days in and we have yet to shut off the engines. Every day the wind dies down to nothing and every night it slowly picks up to five knots on the nose. Flat seas, sun, and sweat seem to be what this passage is all about.

We catch and release two tuna per day; and then I give up trying to catch anything else, though today we actually caught a small shark about two feet long. We got him on the back step and he went nuts, spitting out the lure and thrashing around. I tried to pick him up by the tail; but as I did he arched around 180 degrees trying to take a chomp out of my arm, so I threw him back in. Apparently he didn't want his picture taken.

To pass the time we've been lying on the couch reading, talking to the Australian Coast Watch as they fly past to check us out, and cutting my hair, which has become our new favorite time killer.

Our progress has been excruciatingly slow with currents up to three knots rushing against us. Day one, about a hundred miles from land, we were motoring over a shallow area when our speed suddenly dropped down to one knot. For the next five hours we puttered along like that.

It was brutal, but we figured once the tide turned we would get the current to run with us. Wrong. Eventually the tide did turn but there was no favorable current to go along with it. The rest of the trip has gone pretty much the same way, and now we're not sure how our fuel is going to hold up at this point.

OCTOBER 10, 2005: ASHMORE REEF, AUSRALIA

Some days I just cannot believe where we are or how we ended up here. Today is one of those days. At the moment we are tied up to a mooring hundreds of miles out in the Indian Ocean with not another soul in sight.

This afternoon, after motoring for 114 hours straight, we arrived at Ashmore Reef. We did have a sail up now and then, but the wind was so light it really wasn't any help.

Ashmore Reef is Australian, and they maintain a few heavy duty moorings out here. We tied up and then dropped the dinghy in to cruise over to the shallow water for a swim. This really is an incredible, secluded place.

Of course as I write this and rave about how great and secluded it is, who should appear on the horizon but an Australian customs ship. No doubt they'll come and tie up right next to us and then stare at us with binoculars the rest of the day. It just wouldn't be a proper anchorage otherwise.

An hour after writing about the customs ship arriving, they came over to visit us. And they brought along a film crew. They were filming a show called *Border Security*, following customs officers as they go about their business. They asked us if we would mind if they did a little filming to which we told them that they would have to talk to our agent first. Then we realized that the Post-It note that says, Get Agent, is still on our fridge. So we just welcomed them aboard instead.

OCTOBER 12, 2005: ASHMORE REEF, AUSTRALIA

Right after customs told us that they have a boat posted here 365 days a year, they left, and we've had the place to ourselves ever since. The setting is amazing, being hundreds of miles out at sea, yet surrounded by reef. I don't know how idyllic it would be if the wind picked up, but that doesn't seem very likely as we haven't had wind over five knots for a week now.

The snorkeling has been great and we have seen a little of everything: stingrays, spotted eagle rays, sea snakes, sea turtles, sharks, and loads of fish.

We have slipped into a routine, doing a little boat work in the morning before it gets too hot, and lying around trying not to move in the heat of the afternoon. Then a late afternoon snorkel, followed by a lazy float with the foam noodles in the sandy shallow water, before finally heading back to the boat around five when it starts to cool down. This is going to be one of those places we have to force ourselves to leave.

OCTOBER 14, 2005: EN ROUTE TO INDONESIA

After five incredible days, we finally convinced ourselves that we should really get on our way again. This morning as we were getting ready to go, a customs ship cruised up to the outer reef. As we motored past him, we were hailed on the VHF and asked a few questions.

It's crazy how often these guys ask the same things. Since leaving Darwin we have given our information five times, either to ships or the planes which flew over the reef daily. Only one time have they came back to us, after hearing our boat name, and said they already had all of our information.

Our dinghy has a leak once again. The seams continue to give way one after another. At this point the entire thing is held together with caulk and super glue. I haven't found this latest leak; so until I do, I continue to pump up the dinghy twice a day. If it is left flat, it just swings around violently as we sail.

Yes, sailing. For the first time on our trip to Bali, we have the engines off. There isn't much wind, but we've finally got a favorable current that has helped get our speed up over four knots. Better speeds than the entire first half of the trip. The remainder of this passage should take five days, and I figure we have enough diesel for three. So we can definitely use some good sailing weather.

OCTOBER 16, 2005: EN ROUTE TO INDONESIA

Our slow passage continues. However we are making progress and have managed to sail quite a bit. We are just about in motoring range now. A very good thing, too, as I think if we had to bob around out here waiting for wind we would go insane. The heat is unbearable.

About the only interesting thing to happen has been that our autopilot isn't working properly. Actually it isn't the autopilot so much as the GPS. Normally the GPS gives us a reading within ten feet of where we actually are, but the last couple of days it has been as far off as a quarter of a mile. We've also been hovering eighty feet above sea level which is a really neat trick in a sailboat.

OCTOBER 18, 2005: EN ROUTE TO INDONESIA

The wind has kept up the past couple of days, which has been nice, but the huge thunderstorms that came along with it we could have done without. During one storm it was raining so hard we couldn't see ten feet in front of us. The wind helped us make some mileage though, and it looked like we were going to make it in a night earlier than we had predicted.

This morning we only had forty miles to go. Now eight hours later, we still have twenty-two miles to go. Yes, we have covered a grand total of eighteen miles in the last eight hours. And that's with us motoring. The currents running between the islands of Lombok and Bali are intense and certainly aren't helping us out any. It now looks like we won't be making it in until sometime after midnight.

We are pretty much going crazy with anticipation right now. The last day or two of a long passage is always hard because we get so anxious to get off the boat. Our cooking skills go from being below average to non-existent. Last night, for instance, we had peanut butter toast for dinner. We followed that up this morning with a bowl of potato and bacon soup. We really need to get off of the boat. If for no other reason than to eat a decent meal.

WHEN WE LEFT DARWIN we were pretty happy with ourselves for getting so much boat work done. We had it in our heads that Bali would be a relaxing stop and we wouldn't have to do any work. But this morning Ali updated the Bali to-do list. It includes patching the dinghy leak, fixing the fridge which hasn't shut off since we left Oz, changing the engine oil, having a small tear in the screecher repaired, sanding the cockpit gelcoat repairs that I made in Darwin, making some gelcoat repairs in the galley, cleaning the leather couch before the mold takes over, and applying teak oil to the floors to make them look pretty. Oh, and have fun in Bali. It's ridiculous how much work boats are.

OCTOBER 19, 2005: BALI, INDONESIA

Another 1000-mile passage in the bag. Yesterday was one very long day, but at midnight we crept into the entrance to Bali Marina. The marina is about a mile in from the ocean, and both of our cruising guides warned that we should not attempt a night entrance.

However, we were exhausted at that point and there was no way we were going to stay out all night to wait for the sunrise. Fortunately there was no wind, the water didn't have a ripple on it, and we had a full moon. All things that made a night entry seem perfectly feasible.

We slowed the boat down to two knots and inched our way in. Ali stayed below keeping a close eye on the charts and yelling up directions while I tried to make sense of the navigation lights. The charts actually turned out to be completely inaccurate and showed us motoring across a reef and directly over numerous buoys, but visibility was so good that we didn't need them, and soon we were at the marina. There was a long outer wall and we decided to just tie up there for the night. As we approached it, a couple of marina security guards ran down the dock, grabbed our lines, and helped us get in. Five minutes later we were asleep.

OUR TIME IN BALI was terrific. Back in Australia, Ali and I had started to feel a little burnt out with sailing. Darwin gave us a bit of relief from that, but we were constantly on the go. The passage across to Bali, though, turned out to be one of our best. True, it was hot, and we did very little sailing during those long days, but it was peaceful out on the water. The ocean was smooth for days on end, and we didn't have to give much thought to anything other than if we'd have enough diesel to get us there. And after our time at Ashmore Reef, we were fully recharged.

Then we got to Bali. Man, what a great place. Fantastic people, stunning scenery, and rock bottom prices. What more could a person want? The boat was tied up securely in a dilapidated, yet very well run marina, and we were free to explore the island.

Kuta beach is usually overrun with tourists, but because of the recent bombings most had flown home. We rented a beautiful room just down the street from the beach for next to nothing, and spent a lot of time surfing, lying in the sun, drinking beer, and eating incredible food. This place was our idea of paradise. Once we'd had enough down time on the beach, we rented a car and took off to explore the rest of the island.

One day while driving around, we came across a stretch of road that was covered for miles and miles with woodcarving shops. We stopped and had a look around a few of them. In most we could stand and watch as the person inside carved elaborate masks, furniture, or even a stack of knick knacks you would find at Wal-Mart with a Made in Indonesia sticker on the bottom. Then at once we both spotted a hand-carved wooden rocking horse. It was beautiful, intricate, and way too large a souvenir for somebody living on a boat. But that didn't matter, in no time we'd haggled, reached a deal, and wedged our new horse into the back of our Suzuki Samurai.

OCTOBER 28, 2005: BALI, INDONESIA

At the hotel we had a small crowd gather around to look at our new wooden horse. Everybody seemed really impressed by it and asked us where we got it. One lady asked us if we got it in Bali, which we thought was a pretty funny question. As if we might have brought it with us from America.

Parked out front of a restaurant, a couple of guys stopped to have a look at it. Then one of them came over and asked us if that was our car. He told us what a nice horse it was and asked us where we bought it. Then like everyone else he asked us how much it cost. Instead of answering, we asked him what he thought it would have cost us. He said it must have been over 200,000 rupiah.

Since we were already pretty happy with our purchase and all the attention it brought us, we were glad to hear that we even got it for a good price. We would have never guessed the horse would be such a big hit with the locals.

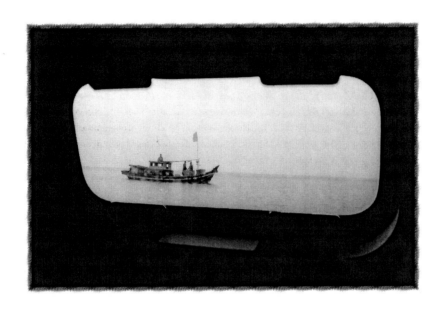

NOVEMBER 8, 2005: BALI, INDONESIA

Today we finished getting ready to leave for Malaysia. We hired a cab to drive us around and finish our shopping list. The first stop was to buy three plastic containers so we could carry another fifteen gallons of diesel onboard. Then to Bali Deli, where it turns out all the ex-patriots go. It's a little store jam packed full of foods from home, wherever home may be. There were bratwursts direct from Germany, spicy Mexican sausages, and my favorite, Cool Ranch Doritos direct from the mighty U.S. of A. Row after row of foods we hadn't seen in two years. We loaded up entirely on snack food, or what some might call junk food, for the passage.

Back at the boat, I found the dinghy completely deflated once again. The thing is really in sad shape. It appears we should have invested in a dinghy cover before the trip. I pumped it back up and quickly tracked down the new leak. I pulled out the dinghy first aid kit, i.e. super glue, and applied my magic touch. Again.

NOVEMBER 9, 2005: EN ROUTE TO MALAYSIA

With the new diesel jugs onboard we are now carrying 110 gallons, something I am very excited about. While sailing we can have too much wind, but I don't think it is possible to ever have too much diesel.

There was a big oil spill in the marina yesterday when one of the large intra-island cruise ships dropped a fifty gallon drum of oil in the water. In no time at all, the oil was everywhere. The marina jumped into action with its emergency plan, which consisted of a very old man using a broken-down rake to sort of push the oil into one corner of the dock. From there he could then scoop it out with a plastic jug. Crisis averted. We spent a couple hours giving the boat a good wash and trying to clean some of the black goo off our hulls.

This morning we headed into the office to pay our bill and collect our passports. Since we aren't planning on stopping anywhere else in Indonesia we cleared out here. The other cruisers were all clearing out in Batam which is just across from Singapore. They said that it should be much easier to clear out there. But instead we just told the marina that we wanted to clear out, and they took care of everything. We never saw an official, and yet this morning our passports had our exit stamps and we had our clearance papers. Piece of cake.

Bum was pretty well hemmed in by a big sailboat on one side and a whole line of small powerboats with nasty outboard props sticking out on the other. Visions of thirty-five foot gel coat scratches danced in our heads, but we managed to get out of our slip without any problems.

After that we negotiated our way through the channel leading back out to the ocean. As we were leaving I became even more impressed with our midnight arrival three weeks earlier. The smallest mistake in this pass and we would have been on a reef.

TODAY'S SAIL WENT PRETTY WELL. We caught the tide and were flying along in ten knots of wind. In the evening, we got to the northeast tip of the island where we found Indonesian fishing boats lining the horizon. I counted 180 of the small boats on the water. We could also see that there were hundreds more pulled up on the beaches. Quite a few of the boats sailed right up alongside of us. The men would smile, wave, and take off again.

Right before dark the wind suddenly picked up to thirty knots, and we were once again caught with the screecher out and no way to get it rolled up. We put out the jib to try and block the wind but that didn't help much. Eventually we decided to furl it the best we could and then release the halyard to drop the whole sail onto the trampolines. It should be easy to yank it back up when we have light winds again.

We've hardly seen any wind since leaving Australia, and the forecast for the next four days shows nothing over ten knots, so we were surprised by this little burst. Almost as soon as we got the sail down the wind began to lighten up, but now two hours later it is howling again. We shouldn't be complaining though as we've got over 1200 miles to go.

NOVEMBER 10, 2005: EN ROUTE TO MALAYSIA
As expected, the wind died down overnight, and by morning it was gone. Ali watched the sun come up and was frightened by what she saw. All around us, some close, some far away, were hundreds of fishing boats. After dark last night we saw just one, by moonlight. So we spent the night sailing in blissful ignorance of just how many boats were actually out there. We were pretty sure the fishermen would be working throughout the night and would make a point of staying out of our way, but then we saw these other things.

There were huge floating rafts all over the place. Fifteen by ten-foot log platforms with a few poles made up into a teepee looking structure, some with a little white flag flapping on top. These seem to be what the fishing nets are attached to. We passed pretty close to one and could see at least three large nets flowing off the back of it, presumably attached to the other raft we could see floating about a quarter mile away. We sailed right past dozens of these this morning, having to alter course more than once. We have no idea how we missed them overnight.

Ali woke me up early this morning to try and decipher what a fisherman was trying to say. He was waving his arm to direct us away from his nets but it was impossible to tell which way he was trying to point us. We would think it would be universally understood how to point somebody in a direction, but his arm movements had us bewildered. Eventually he took off ahead of us in his boat and we followed him. Once he seemed sure that we wouldn't do something stupid, like run over his nets, he circled around and went back to work.

Ali mentioned how easy it would have been for us to hit something in the night out here. I tried to convince her that the odds of us running into anything in this great big ocean were nearly zilch. But after seeing all the crap floating around this morning, I'm not so sure I believe myself any more.

With no wind this morning we took the opportunity to get the screecher sail back up. Now hopefully we'll see a little bit of wind so we can use it.

NOVEMBER 12, 2005: EN ROUTE TO MALAYSIA

This is shaping up to be the slowest passage ever for *Bumfuzzle*. We have yet to make even a one-hundred-mile day. That's slow.

Yesterday we had light winds on the nose. Combined with a current of one to two knots against us we were barely moving. We kept expecting the current to change along with the tide, but after a dropping tide, slack water, and a rising tide, we still couldn't get the boat going over three knots. Eventually I decided to stop the boat, jump in to have a look underneath, and make sure we weren't dragging a fishing net. We weren't, but I wish we had been.

We spent the day once again dodging fishing obstacles. Now instead of rafts with teepees on them, we've got rafts with just a tiny flag on top in different colors so the fishermen can identify them. The rafts are virtually impossible to see during the day and in the dark we are flying blind.

Last night during my first watch, I was sitting in the cockpit when I suddenly saw a flag go floating by just inches from the side of the boat. I jumped up and braced myself for some sort of impact or at least for the boat to suddenly drag to a stop from catching a line of nets, but somehow we missed everything.

Ali's watches were uneventful until this morning when a boat with ten men aboard began following us. We've had a lot of boats cruise close to us in order to satisfy their curiosity, but this one was different. They were crossing adjacent to us a hundred yards back but then turned straight behind us and closed to about fifty yards, where they continued to follow along slowly.

After a few minutes she woke me to have a look. I had to agree it was pretty strange. We were sailing very slowly in light winds, so we decided to start the engines, increase our speed, and see what they would do. Five minutes after we sped up, they turned off and continued the way they were originally going. I'm sure it was nothing, it just seemed weird.

Today things went a little better. Our speed was still ridiculously slow but we were at least able to sail most of the time. In order for us to make it to Malaysia we will need to sail four out of the twelve hundred miles. So far we've managed one hundred. If that doesn't improve soon we'll need to get more diesel somewhere along the way.

I KNOW FROM WATCHING MOVIES and reading books it sounds as if every day at sea is a battle against mountainous waves and terrible storms, but the reality, at least ninety-five percent of the time, is much different. Here is an example of our typical day on passage.

"A day in the life of *Bumfuzzle* at sea"

7 - 10 p.m. Ali is sleeping, and I am on watch staring out into the darkness while waiting for the inevitable impact of a floating Gilligan's Island hut. Doing so has caused me to ponder why they don't put headlights on boats. I'm also listening to *A Year In*

Provence on the iPod and have decided there is nothing more lame than listening to a Frenchman talk about French food. Except of course listening to Ali and I talk about the Taco Bell menu after a few days at sea. Mmmm, grilled stuffed burritos.

10 - 1 a.m. Ali's watch. She spends it reading, writing e-mails, and sticking her head outside every five minutes to make sure we aren't going to run over any fishing boats, or miscellaneous rafts. Right at the end of her watch the wind finally picks up enough for us to roll out the screecher sail.

1 - 4 a.m. My watch again. This time I emptied our three new diesel containers into the tanks, wrote a couple of e-mails, played a little poker on the computer, and sat outside anxiously awaiting the end of a very boring audio book while trying desperately to stay awake.

4 - 8 a.m. Ali's watch. There is nothing to do but read and write a few more e-mails. At six she wakes me to keep an eye on the mystery boat. I go back to bed while she downloads and reads new e-mail.

8:30 a.m. Ali goes back to bed while I try to wake up. Have an apple, a glass of water, and read e-mail. Then I sit outside weaving my way through the fishing nets that are scattered all over the place. At least it is still cool enough to sit outside.

10 a.m. Ali is up and it's time for a snack. Some pretzels and a can of pop. We both lie on the couch reading, and take turns having a look around outside every few minutes.

12 p.m. More snacking, because there is nothing else to do. How about some more pretzels and a hunk of spicy Mexican sausage? Yum. Funny thing is that we really enjoy it and start to talk about how we should have bought four more of the sausages and at least a couple more bags of pretzels. Then we realize we might be getting delirious when we start discussing the merits of pretzels and where they rank in the snack food hall of fame. It is so hot that we sweat just turning the pages of our books, so we continue lying around, trying not to do anything but survive the heat.

1:15 - 1:18 p.m. Read *Sail* magazine. Find that there is nothing but articles about racing and safety. It does nothing to help alleviate my boredom. I make a mental note not to read about sailing while I'm actually sailing. Now I remember why we didn't renew our subscriptions to a single magazine.

2:00 p.m. Frustrated with the state of the sailing magazine industry, I sit down at the computer and bang out an article that is in no way related to racing or safety at sea. I proofread it and realize that if I submitted it I would just be contributing even more to the dullness that defines the sailing magazine. Delete article. Ali is sweating and staring blankly at the ceiling. I debate whether or not to give her our last can of Sweat cola from Bali, but decide it is too early on in the trip.

2:15 p.m. The wind is gone again. We roll up the screecher.

3 - 4 p.m. Now we are getting excited. This is the time of day when the heat has topped out and it starts to gradually cool down. We sit outside in the shade and wait, and wait, and wait. The wind is back, but barely. We put the screecher out again.

4 p.m. Dinner time. Ali's not feeling so good so I don't get a full-on gourmet meal. It's alright though, it is probably best not to have chili dogs three nights in a row. Instead tonight's meal is a can of soup and some bread. Delicious. Best of all is that the whole meal took five minutes to make and only made one pot dirty. To us, those two things form the basis of any good meal. Describing even that simple meal would have taken Peter Mayle six pages. I hate Peter Mayle, and after listening to his book I now feel an unnerving prejudice towards the French.

4:15 p.m. The wind disappears so we roll the screecher back in.

4:30 p.m. Finally cool enough to shower. It's a fine line because if we shower too early we will be wallowing in our own sweat again and all will be lost. But we can't wait too long because we are so excited to be clean and refreshed.

5:30 p.m. We are motoring and the sea is smooth. Ideal conditions for still more lying on the couch, only now we are clean and not sweating at all. We eat some weird cookies from Holland. They're pretty good, but I think they are called biscuits over there and are supposed to be eaten with tea. I dunk mine in cherry Kool-Aid instead.

6:30 p.m. Back outside for the best half hour of the day. It's cool outside and we sit next to each other watching another beautiful sunset. We have the discussion about how many days we have been at sea and how many more are left until we get where we are going. Usually this conversation doesn't come up until after the midway point of the trip, but this time we've only made it a third of the way. Not a good sign.

7:00 p.m. Ali leaves me for her three hours of blissful sleep and I sit at the computer typing this.

Repeat.

That's it, our day at sea. Obviously things are a little different when there are strong winds, but not nearly as much as one might think. In fact this day was probably more active than most since there was so much crap floating in the water for us to watch out for. On a normal passage we can easily go twenty minutes between looking around. Here in Indonesian waters we have had to be much more alert. So anyway, that was a pretty typical day for us as we slowly make our way from one great place to the next.

It always makes us laugh when people who haven't been out here like this tell us how much they are going to enjoy the solitude when they do go sailing. They talk about how they are going to teach themselves Spanish, how to play the guitar, and to cook French pastries. Maybe they're right and we're just weird, but on passages we just can't get motivated to do much of anything.

One thing we really find hard to believe is that cruisers spend all day preparing and cooking meals during passages. That is all the cruising books talk about. We just cannot imagine it. For one thing we just don't have much of an appetite, and for another, who has the energy?

NOVEMBER 15, 2005: EN ROUTE TO MALAYSIA

I just wrote an entire paragraph about the last three days but after reading it through I realized that it can all be summed up in one sentence; there is nothing going on out here. That's really all that needs to be said, but I'll say more anyway.

There is little to no wind, flat seas, very few ships or fishing boats, no more of those fishing net structures, a couple of dolphins who have managed to survive all the fishing nets, a few disgusting yellow sea snakes, a ton of broken up pieces of styrofoam, and that is it. It's not all bad though, at night when we are sailing along at a super slow three knots with no waves slapping against the boat we sleep like babies. Staying awake during our watches is the hard part.

NOVEMBER 18, 2005: EN ROUTE TO MALAYSIA

We continue to move along at a blistering pace, with an average speed now of close to 3.75 knots. Today we were lying out in the sun, motoring headlong into a two-knot current, when Ali suddenly said, "We can't even say we're sailing around the world. We're just going around the world on a boat."

What she meant is that we never seem to sail, we are always motoring. My advice to anybody going out to sail around the world would be to carry at least twice as much diesel as they think necessary. And the upgraded, larger engines probably wouldn't be a bad idea either.

Her comment got me to thinking about when I was planning our first big crossing, from the Bahamas to Panama. I calculated the mileage and then figured out how long it would take at an average speed of five, six, or seven knots. At the time I thought that five knots would be the absolute slowest speed that we could average. Now, after a whole lot of passages, I realize that we have only averaged better than five knots twice. I use four knots as my trip planning speed now, and even that seems to be a reach most of the time.

The last few days have been extremely uneventful. We did manage to sail for a couple of days, albeit very slowly in light winds. It was enough, however, that I began to think we were within motoring range of our destination, which is a good thing because the wind has completely abandoned us again.

Yesterday while motoring between a couple islands, we decided to pull over for the afternoon. Nice thing out here is that we can anchor pretty much anywhere because it is so shallow. We dropped the anchor about two miles out from land in forty feet of water and got some much needed rest. Even on an easy passage like this we find ourselves exhausted after a few days, and it feels really good to not have to worry about anything for a few hours.

We thought for sure that we'd be visited by fishermen at some point during the day but nobody ever came anywhere near us. Surprisingly to me, other than the occasional holler and wave, we don't seem to arouse much interest from the small fishing boats.

Around seven o'clock, the tide had turned and the current let up, so we hauled in the anchor and headed out again. We have had some really nice night watches lately with a full moon and cooler temps. In fact last night was the first time I've put a shirt on since we left Bali over a week ago.

Right now we are motoring through an area about which our cruising guide says, "Recent news suggests avoiding Selat Bangka, especially at night." And that's all it says. It doesn't say what that recent news was, or why we are supposed to avoid this particular area. It seems that no matter what, you just cannot avoid the pirate threats. We've only got 100 miles to go until the infamous Malacca Straits. Home of Blackbeard and Captain Hook I think. But I'm not sure, I'm not really up on my pirates.

NOVEMBER 20, 2005: EN ROUTE TO MALAYSIA

The sky off to our west was really dark today and Ali thought it looked like we were going to get rain. I said, "Nah, the wind is coming from the east, that should be moving away from us."

Within half an hour the clouds were on top of us. The lower layer of clouds looked as if they were right on the water, and we could see them clearly as they rolled over and over themselves approaching us. We closed the hatches, dropped the main, rolled in the jib, and made sure everything else was secure. It was obvious we were about to get blasted.

Then a hundred yards away we could see the waves appear like magic out of the calm water. Seconds later, we felt a swirling gust of cold air as the wind went from the east at ten knots to the west at twenty-five.

That turned out to be as bad as the wind got though, and within a few minutes we were putting up sail. While I was standing in the rain at the wheel, I had a little bird come join me. These guys always seem to appear out of nowhere when the weather turns ugly. This one flew right under the bimini and landed eighteen inches in front of my face. He then moved over into the cockpit and laid himself out flat. We uncoiled a jib line next to him and he soon made himself a little nest in it. At first light, as they always do, he gave a little tweet and flew off.

Gradually the wind died and we went back to motoring. Throughout the night our speed continued to plummet until we were only moving at one knot. I was searching the charts for some solution. We were ten miles from land and our options seemed pretty limited. But seeing as the seas were pretty calm, there hadn't been much shipping traffic, and the water was only eighty feet deep, I decided to wake Ali up and drop the anchor.

It was strange to be anchored so far from land with nothing protecting us. Even stranger was that it felt like we were anchored in the middle of a raging river. The current was running over three knots and kept the boat bucking against the anchor chain the rest of the night, during which time we continued our watches to make sure that we weren't run down by a ship while we slept.

After a few hours, the current had let up and we took off again. Two miles farther on, we sailed over the equator putting us back in the northern hemisphere where we'll stay for the rest of our trip.

THIS AFTERNOON ALI WAS OUTSIDE trying to avoid all the crap in the water, and I was down below trying to get some sleep when I suddenly felt a vibration in the engine. I went outside and found Ali looking over the side of the boat. We shut down the engine and she said that there had just been a long line of garbage in the water that she could not avoid.

We see these occasionally out at sea, garbage caught in a current and stretching for miles. Knowing we must have snagged something in the prop, I put on my goggles and stuck my head in the water. I couldn't see a thing, the water was the color of coffee with milk. We were only about four hours from where we had decided to anchor for the night, so we decided to leave it until we got there and just use the other engine in the meantime.

That was going well until the current kicked back in and we really needed both engines to keep us moving. We stopped the boat and I jumped in. I couldn't even see my hand in front of my face and had to just feel my way around the bottom of the boat blindly. I found the prop and grabbed hold of a big plastic bag wrapped up around it. Fortunately it hadn't gotten too tangled up and I was able to quickly pull it free and get us back underway.

Just as we were approaching our anchorage for the night, the skies opened up again to make sure that we were thoroughly soaked during the anchoring process.

NOVEMBER 21, 2005: EN ROUTE TO MALAYSIA

After anchoring last night we settled in, had dinner, did dishes, and worked on the computer. Then right before dark a boat came puttering up alongside of us. I went outside to say hello and found three guys on a wooden fishing boat hanging on to the side of our boat. I smiled and tried to make conversation but they acted like I wasn't even there, not making eye contact, and trying to look around our boat. Eventually they moved towards the stern where they could get a good look in the cockpit door.

The three of them sat staring and talking amongst themselves for what felt like forever while I smiled and tried to act friendly. They continued to ignore me until one of them climbed onto our back transom and began walking towards the cockpit. Still trying to act nice, I made hand gestures in front of him indicating I wanted him off the boat. Ali also stepped out into the cockpit looking pissed. He turned and talked with one of the other guys and then climbed back onto his boat. Without a wave or saying a word they motored slowly around the boat and headed towards shore.

It was a weird experience and we didn't feel like it was at all friendly or even just locals being curious. It felt a lot more like we were being scoped out. We knew that there was no way we would be able to get a good night of sleep there, so we decided to get moving again instead. Within minutes we had the anchor up and were on our way. The wind was in our favor for a change and we zipped along at seven knots for a couple of hours until we were well away from the area.

Around midnight the wind disappeared and the current set against us. We decided once again to pull into shallow water and anchor. Fortunately this time nothing strange happened and we were able to get a few hours of rest.

By six o'clock the current had spun around and we were moving again. Almost as soon as we raised the anchor it began to pour. The rain didn't let up the rest of the morning while we dodged between fishing boats and what looked like huge oil rig platforms. A few hours later, like clockwork, we were once again stopped dead in our tracks by the current.

We are cutting it very close with diesel, so whenever our speed drops below two knots we have to stop and wait it out. It's slow going this way, but at least we are getting more sleep.

We continued the start and stop routine throughout the day until strong winds and a lack of shelter forced us to seek an alternative. I had a look at the charts and found an island about ten miles away that we could hide behind for the night. The only problem with this place was that it would take us right next to the main shipping channel. Now instead of crossing the Malacca Strait up north near Port Klang, we would have to cross it to the south right around the corner from Singapore.

NOVEMBER 22, 2005: EN ROUTE TO MALAYSIA

What a day. We managed a whopping twenty-four miles. This morning we woke up to the fourth day in a row of pure ugliness. The sky has been a solid dark gray sheet that sits on top of the murky brown water. After a few hours of waiting for the weather to clear, we gave up and decided we'd go cross the Malacca Strait, the busiest shipping channel in the world. Why not, we had nothing else to do.

We motored out from behind our little island and found conditions just about as bad as the day before. We motorsailed into the wind for a couple of hours until it was time to make our turn and cross the shipping lanes. There was a pretty steady stream of ships going in each direction, but we found an opening and sailed into it. We just made it through the southbound traffic before the biggest container ship we've ever seen charged past us.

In between the lanes there is a "median" a couple of hundred yards wide. This area was covered with local fishing boats with their scattering of nets all over the place. Negotiating the nets was more of a hazard than the ships.

We waited in the middle while three ships cruised by, and then finished the last couple of miles without incident. Definitely not something we would like to do at night, but it wasn't bad during the day when we could see clearly just how far away the ships were. We were happy for the well-charted shipping lanes and for the fact that the ships actually stay in between them.

Once on the other side, we were basically out of sailing room; and with the strong headwind, we were pretty well screwed as far as getting anywhere the rest of the day. Fortunately there was an island nearby which we could tuck in behind, and that's where we are now after our twenty-four-mile day.

We are really in about the worst state of mind that we have ever been in on this trip. Even allowing for a very slow passage, my worst case scenario was twelve days. Now fourteen days in we are still a minimum of two days away. That is a ridiculous amount of time to cover just 1200 miles. Brutal. We should have bought a speedboat.

NOVEMBER 24, 2005: EN ROUTE TO MALAYSIA

Seventy miles to go. It looks like we might make it after all, although it is going to be a close call. Our diesel situation is dire, but by my calculations we should make it with three gallons to spare.

The weather calmed throughout the night, and by two a.m. we could see a few stars and the moon for the first time in a week. When we woke up this morning the weather had magically transformed to what it was before all this rain came along, ninety-five degrees, sunny, and calm. Hopefully it holds out one more night and allows us to limp into Port Klang, tired and wet.

Today is Thanksgiving. Now there is a holiday that doesn't travel very well around the world. Needless to say there will be no turkey and stuffing onboard *Bum* tonight. The fridge is officially empty. We are out of bread, fruit, vegetables, and meat, which does not leave a whole lot to work with for a Thanksgiving feast. We'll be having soup and crackers for dinner.

NOVEMBER 25, 2005: PORT KLANG, MALAYSIA

Malaysia at last. Wow was that a long passage. Sixteen days to cover only twelve hundred miles. That's got to be some sort of record. There were a few times out there that I really felt like slamming my head into a wall. Ali did pretty well, since she had gotten all of her frustration out of her system within the first six days of the passage.

The weather wasn't great, especially the last week, but the currents were the real killer, keeping us down at an average speed of only three knots. But hey, it's over, and now we're only a three-day sail from Thailand. That sounds like nothing to us now. It'll be like going down the street to pick up milk.

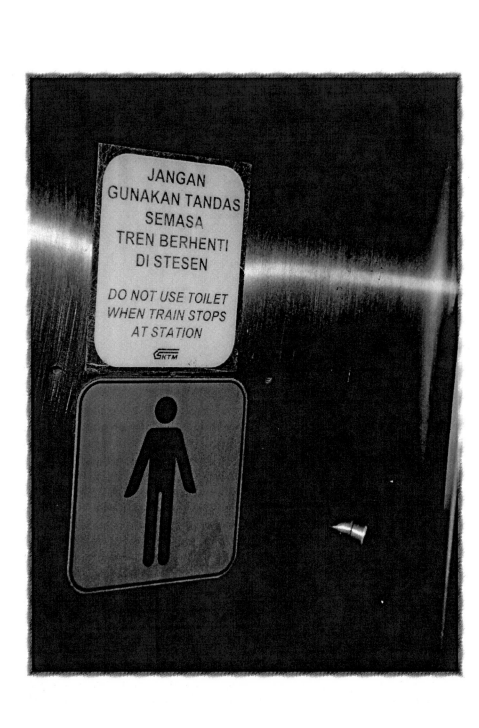

these guys are professionals

DECEMBER 5, 2005: PORT KLANG, MALAYSIA

During the past few days we've covered some miles. The difference is that this time we have done it on the trains. We visited Kuala Lumpur but didn't find much of interest there, so we continued on to Singapore. This was a more interesting city, especially the neighborhoods on the outskirts of the main downtown area. We hit a few of the tourist sites there and then made our way back to the boat. We're usually big city lovers, but right now we've got visions of Thailand on the mind.

This morning we woke up with every intention of leaving today. But after washing the boat, walking into town to clear customs and immigration, and picking up the laundry, we just didn't have the energy to go sailing. We're out of here in the morning.

DECEMBER 6, 2005: PORT KLANG, MALAYSIA

It's one a.m., we're tied to a dock, and we just came as close to sinking as we ever hope to again. At eleven o'clock Ali and I finished up some work we were doing on the internet and walked back down to the boat.

The dock we are tied up to is just sixty yards downstream from a very busy shipping dock. The boats that use that dock are large Indonesian wooden cargo ships used to haul goods back and forth between Malaysia and the nearby Indonesian islands. The boats have one engine and no bow thrusters, so when they need to maneuver, things can get a little crazy. Especially on the falling tide when the current is running at five knots down river.

Anyway, we had just gotten back on the boat and watched as one of these cargo ships performed a wild full-speed spin heading downstream with the current. I knew he was just turning around so that he could pull into the docks facing into the current so I didn't think too much of it. Ali started brushing her teeth and I was downstairs using the bathroom when I suddenly heard an engine revving at full throttle. It sounded like it was right on top of us, but I wasn't sure because down in the hulls noises always sound amplified. Seconds later there was a sickening crunch.

I zipped up and ran outside to find Ali already on deck yelling at the top of her lungs. I looked forward and saw the bow of the boat that had been docked in front of us was now crashing into us, having been nailed by the huge cargo ship we'd been watching minutes earlier. Our front dockline and our forward spring line had both snapped from the pressure and our boat was trying to peel itself off the dock with the force of the current and the other boat pressing against us. I made a jump for the dock but didn't make it and slammed down into the skanky water before Ali and I quickly got another line tied off to the bow.

About this time the German single-hander from the boat that was on top of ours came walking casually down the dock, seemingly oblivious as to what was happening. Ali began screaming at him to back his boat off of ours.

Eventually he started backing up, but we had to stop him because his anchor was snagged on our lifeline and his boat couldn't move backwards without ripping our boat apart. A Malaysian guy jumped on our boat and the three of us managed to lift the bow of the German boat enough to get his anchor unhooked and the boat began backing away from us. We quickly got a couple more lines tied off and our boat seemed secure. All of this took about four minutes of frantic screaming and maneuvering.

We started to assess the damage, but could see right away that we had been extremely fortunate. Our boats had been facing each other and somehow his boat managed to slam into ours in about the only spot that it wouldn't destroy us. His bow missed the front of our starboard bow by about a foot and instead hit the lifelines and the huge metal brace that runs between our bows.

By now a few people were out on the dock helping the German with his lines. Ali and I figured things were under control, but then things got even crazier. I noticed the German was having trouble getting his boat tied up properly again, and walked over to help. I adjusted a couple of the front lines and then Ali started yelling from the front of our boat that his boat was going to hit ours again. I looked over and saw the German desperately pulling the middle spring line while the back of his boat was floating quickly away from the dock.

I couldn't believe what was happening. Things had been fine seconds earlier and everybody had begun slowly dispersing. Now here I'll mention that the German had been up at the bar when this all started and he'd been drinking for a few hours. Obviously there's nothing wrong with that, it just kind of makes some of his actions a little clearer.

So here we now have a skinny drunk man trying to hold his boat in place while a five knot current spins the back end off of the dock. I ran past him to the two back lines to get them tightened before the back of the boat swung all the way around and smashed into our boat.

I grabbed the first line, which was loose, and started pulling on it quickly to get the slack out before tying it off to the dock. But as I pulled the line it suddenly plopped right into the water. The German had forgotten to tie it off to his boat cleat. There was still one other line, which was as slack as it could go, and it was quickly coming taut. It was tied to a dock cleat that was too far forward and wouldn't keep the boat from spinning around, so I went to untie it to bring it to a dock cleat further back. But the line wasn't just tied off around the cleat, it was tied in a knot through the cleat. I don't know what purpose people have for doing this but it is truly idiotic. I couldn't get the knot undone and seconds later that line came taut with a ton of force behind it.

Now his boat is ninety degrees to the dock and to our boat. It is about ten feet in front of us, sideways to a five knot current, and has one front line and one back line holding it. While I had been trying to get the back lines taken care of, Ali had been absolutely screaming at the German to forget about the line he was holding and to get on his boat. He finally did and was now backing down hard on the engine trying to swing the back of his boat back around towards the dock. Immediately I knew that was hopeless, and yelled to Ali to get me the dive knife.

By this point of the debacle, two cleats had ripped out of the dock, two of our lines and two of the Germans lines had snapped like silly string. It was painfully clear that these last two lines weren't going to hold him. If either of them snapped, our boat would be destroyed, and there was no way that his boat was going to be able to back around into this current. Ali was still on the front of our boat yelling that he was about to hit us, so I made a decision. I yelled to the guy that I was going to cut his lines. He yelled, "Noooooo," apparently thinking he could somehow get it under control. He still had the engine cranked in reverse and I thought it was the only way we could save our boat. So I cut the lines.

It doesn't take much to cut a line that is under that sort of pressure. All I had to do was touch the dive knife to them and they exploded. His 100 horsepower engine blasted the boat straight back perpendicular to our bow while Ali and I held our breath. Honestly, he missed ripping our port bow apart by less than a foot. Ali stood there inches away while his anchor and bow swung directly over the top of ours. It was unbelievable.

At last the German seemed to be safely away from the dock and out of our hair. But now we looked up to see him racing right back towards us. We're thinking that maybe he is trying to pull back to the same dock he was just at so we yell at him to go around to a much safer inside berth. But he yells back that there is a line tangled in his rudder and he can't steer. What else could go wrong? We watch as he begins floating at five knots right down the middle of the river. Then he quickly ran forward to drop his anchor and, amazingly, the boat swung around and stopped. Finally, everything seemed to be safe.

Ali and I then took a close look at our boat and couldn't believe how lucky we had been. Aside from a couple of bent stanchions, and some minor cracks in the gelcoat, we had escaped major damage. If things had happened just a little differently our trip could have had a very unhappy ending tonight. We might take a lot of risk sailing around in an uninsured boat but we never dreamed we could lose the boat at a dock.

The police eventually showed up, but didn't even talk to us. Not that we really wanted to talk to them. I could just imagine filling out a police report on this incident. Wait, I know, we'll sue. Let's see, an Indonesian cargo ship in Malaysian waters, hits a German boat that then hits our American boat. We're not going to hold our breath and expect a compensation check any time soon.

Alright, it's after two a.m. and I think I've finally calmed down enough to get some sleep. Ali crashed a half an hour ago.

STILL THE SAME DAY, but it feels like it's been a week since last night. Ali woke me up this morning at seven o'clock to tell me that another boat was leaving. I took the hint and said that we should leave too. A half-hour later we quietly slipped away from the dock and floated down the river. We really just wanted to get the heck out of there and weren't the least bit interested in talking to the Malaysian police today, not to mention reliving last night for all of the dock gawkers.

Today my body feels like I've been beaten up. My legs are sore, my arms and legs have cuts on them, and my knuckles are all bruised up. Things got a little intense last night.

Throughout the day we just kept talking about how bad things could have been. For one thing, we had originally been tied up to the dock right where the German got hit. The only reason we had moved forward was because our water hose wasn't long enough to reach the spout and I couldn't wash the boat. Then there is the fact that we had just returned from being away from the boat for five days. We can't even imagine what would have happened if we hadn't been there. A pretty unbelievable set of circumstances caused us to walk away from this one with just a few scratches.

So now we are on passage again. It was the nicest day we've had since we arrived in Malaysia, though not much wind. There were many fishing boats along our route today. They all do a good job of staying out of our way, which is nice since I believe they've actually got the right of way. Despite their boats shabby appearances, these guys are professionals and they don't want us running their nets over any more than we want to, so they make it pretty easy on us.

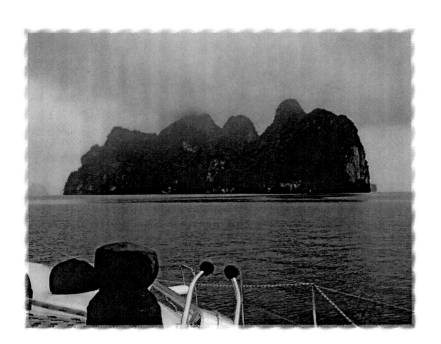

big seas and bigger fish

DECEMBER 7, 2005: EN ROUTE TO THAILAND

We can't wait to be done with the Malacca Straits. No matter what we do we can not get the boat over four knots. There just doesn't seem to be any way to do things quickly out here.

We had a wicked storm raging most of last night. The lightning was striking so close that it burned our eyeballs just like if we were staring right into the sun. Then there was the instantaneous crack of thunder to scare the crap out of us. All the while we had to stand outside in the downpour to keep an eye out for fishing boats. I don't think either one of us felt badly when it came time to wake the other person up for their watch.

DECEMBER 11, 2005: MAYA BAY, THAILAND

This morning the wind shifted a bit, and for the first time in weeks we weren't beating into it on our way north, a welcome relief. When we arrived at Maya Bay on Phi Phi Leh it was pouring down rain, however it did nothing to detract from the beauty of the island.

It was exactly what I had dreamt Thailand would look like, which was a good thing because Thailand is probably the number one stop that we have been looking forward to on this trip. Once again, it is hard for us to comprehend that we've sailed halfway around the world to get here, moored twenty yards from a limestone cliff that soars straight up hundreds of feet above us. It almost seems absurd to think that two years ago we sailed away from Florida without a clue as to what we were doing. And yet here we are. It really makes us laugh to think about it.

I jumped in the water to have my first look at the bottom of the boat since Ashmore Reef. It wasn't pretty. Our port engine prop trailed long tendrils of plastic bag behind it. Over the last couple of days I had noticed that the engine seemed to be about a half knot slower than the starboard engine; but it wasn't overheating and still had good water flow, so I didn't worry about it. Our water line has also developed a real ugliness to it lately because of how filthy the water has been everywhere. Even scrubbing doesn't take it off very easily, but I spent my day doing it anyway.

DECEMBER 14, 2005: MAYA BAY, THAILAND

Well I think we can officially say that we have made it through the Malacca Straits. The famously dangerous pirate-filled waters of the Malacca Straits to be more exact. So I thought now would be a good time to quote what one particularly disgruntled old cruiser had to say in the cruising forums a few months back.

". . . all the hard parts lie ahead, while the Coconut Milk Run has a relatively well-deserved name. My wish for Pat and Ali is that they sail NNW from NZ via Tonga before heading to Oz - certainly not try it straight across the Tasman Sea - and after enjoying the Coral Coast, ship the boat to either the Med or the States, depending on their remaining interest in cruising and the size of their residual kitty.

I'm especially concerned about the Malacca Straits and either the Red Sea or South Africa as sailing grounds for these willing but unskilled sailors. My hunch is that something of this nature - a truncated voyage - will soon look like a reasonable alternative for them."

I just love that, "certainly not try it straight across the Tasman Sea", "especially concerned about the Malacca Straits", ship the boat to the Med or go home because we're out of money. Sorry to disappoint you buddy but it seems your "hunch" was wrong. These two "unskilled sailors", who have only two years and 17,000 miles of sailing behind them, which is certainly not enough, have just completed everything that you said they shouldn't, or couldn't do. What a wimp.

We set out on this trip for the adventure; the adventure of sailing around the world. I want to tell my grandkids really cool stories about big seas and bigger fish. And now I've got a whole warehouse full of those stories. And best of all is that I've got an incredible wife who was standing right next to me through it all and who has shared all of the adventure with me.

As for the internet chat room drones, they'll just never get that and they'll never give us any credit. To them we will always just be the "unskilled sailors" who shouldn't be out here taking on the ocean. Just like them.

I REALLY DON'T UNDERSTAND why it is so hard for so many lifelong sailors to accept that we are doing this. I would have thought that the internet would have created more adventurous people. It certainly did for us. But it seemed that instead what it was doing was giving the naysayers and the lazy a place to gather to talk about why people shouldn't be adventurous. It became a place to list all the reasons not to do something instead of reasons to do it.

There aren't many true adventures left in the world, but no matter how things change this one will always be there. Believe it or not there are still people who think nothing of throwing caution to the wind.

DECEMBER 25, 2005: BANGKOK, THAILAND

It was Christmas Eve and we were in Bangkok on the famous Khao San Road. What better place could there be to give each other a Christmas present? We both decided that this trip had become a big enough part of our lives that it was time to immortalize it. We each wrote bumfuzzle on the other's arm and sat down in the chair to brand ourselves for life. It only seemed logical.

Back out on Khao San afterwards, we pulled up a street side table at a little bar to enjoy the holiday atmosphere. The hawkers were in full swing trying to sell oversize lighters, cheap jewelry, and little toys. There were Christmas decorations, holiday music, and even a skinny Thai Santa who had trouble keeping his pants from falling down. It was an absolutely perfect Christmas Eve.

JANUARY 8, 2006: PHUKET, THAILAND

We just finished reading *Dove*, which is a book that just about every sailing dreamer has already read. It's about a sixteen-year-old kid who sails around the world. I liked some of the book, the sailing and adventure parts, but throughout the book he would also go on and on about how terrible modern society is, and how bland and pointless everybody's life is, except his, because they are working to earn a dollar while he is free as the wind. It's almost like he completely forgot that it was his father whose pointless existence had paid for his boat in the first place.

It's really annoying, but I do understand it. Sometimes it is hard not to feel superior when you are out here living this awesome adventure. We start to wonder why everybody doesn't do it. We have to remind ourselves that not everybody wants to do this sort of thing and that they could be just as happy doing something totally different or ordinary.

A little running around to do today and then we are off. This morning we have to clear out of the country, stop at the post office, and pick up our laundry. After that we're headed for Sri Lanka.

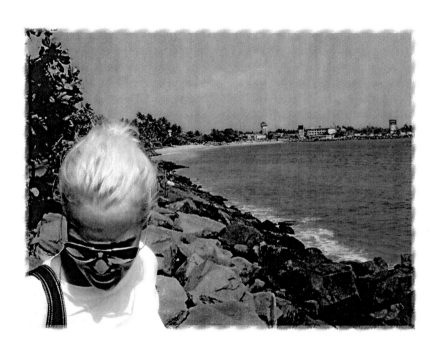

me and Bobbi Jean

WE ENJOYED THAILAND, even if Phuket was way too touristy. The plan had been to spend a lot more time cruising the islands there, but the weather simply would not cooperate with us. So instead, for Christmas, we hopped a flight to Bangkok.

What an awesome city. Walking around it you just felt alive. It was vibrant, always moving, and always different. Around every corner was something new. We visited markets, temples, tattoo parlors, and even attended a rowdy Thai boxing match. To us Bangkok felt like the real Thailand. Though I'm sure the same would be said out in the countryside, where the experience would be nearly the opposite. I guess it is safe to say there is a lot to explore in Thailand, and we hardly scratched the surface.

SOMETHING HAPPENED TO US in Bangkok. Something that changed us for the better and that would affect all of our traveling in the future.

We were wandering around downtown, and must have looked lost when a man approached us. He asked where we were going and then instead of simply pointing us in the right direction he walked along with us for a couple of blocks. Once we were on the right track, he said goodbye and turned back the other way.

When we reached the Grand Palace we stood across the street admiring it. A young guy walked up to us and said hello. He then went through the normal questions of asking us where we were from and what we were doing there, while explaining that he was a student at the university just across the street. By now our radar was up and both of us were wondering just what this guy wanted.

He told us the Grand Palace was closed to visitors since it was Christmas Eve and the King would be spending the holidays there. But, he said, there were plenty of other things to see. He grabbed our map and began circling streets and telling us what was there. Once he finished he flagged down a tuk-tuk, negotiated with the driver to take us all over town, and settled on a price of seventy-five cents. At this point Ali and I are thinking that this guy was very nice but there had to be a catch. We climbed in the tuk-tuk and waited for the scam. But instead he said to us, "Goodbye. I hope you enjoy Thailand. When I am a tourist in America I hope someone will be able to help me out."

The tuk-tuk drove us to all the places that we had highlighted and we had a great time. Every place we visited was something we otherwise would have never seen.

At the end of the day, Ali and I talked about how on guard, and probably sort of rude, we had been with the strangers we met. Yet all anybody had wanted to do was help us out and make sure we enjoyed our visit to their home. We had never been scammed so why did we assume we would be. We made a pact right there and then, that from now on we would only expect the best from people and we would go with the flow. After making that decision our entire trip changed.

JANUARY 14, 2006: SIMILAN ISLANDS, THAILAND

We left Ao Chalong the other day and sailed around the island to Patong Bay. The wind was blowing around thirty knots, but we were sailing right in close to land and avoiding the big waves. Sailing like that can be a little tricky because the wind often drops way down as we are hidden behind land and then gusts suddenly to thirty knots. We had to be careful not to get hit with too much sail up.

After anchoring a long way out from the beach, we caught a few hours of sleep before setting out for the Similan Islands about sixty miles off the coast.

We left at two a.m. in order to make it out to the islands before dark the next day. It was a beautiful night with a full moon, no wind, and total quiet out on the water.

A little after sunrise we had a big pod of dolphins join us. It was nice to see something in the water again. The waters of SE Asia are so busy with fisherman that we had begun to wonder how anything could live through it.

Later in the afternoon, Ali was hanging up a towel to dry when a whale suddenly breached right behind us less than 100 feet away and headed our direction. We stood there and waited for him to resurface, which he did, but this time a little further back. Ali was thrilled to see a whale again, but I was actually hoping we wouldn't see any for a while. It seems every story I have read about boats hitting whales happens in the Indian Ocean. Granted, it would be a cool story, but I'm not sure I feel like testing the strength of our boat on the back of a whale.

We didn't have detailed charts for the Similan Islands and were counting on picking up a mooring when we got there, knowing that it was a huge dive charter destination. However we were still surprised by the huge number of boats that were there, especially since it is a National Park.

There were park service moorings all over the place and we grabbed one just off the island in water over a hundred feet deep. Yet, just fifty feet away it shelved straight up into beautiful light blue water filled with coral. I jumped right in and went snorkeling in what was some of the best coral I've seen anywhere.

This morning we found thousands of bright blue and yellow fish swimming around the back of the boat. Unfortunately the water was disgusting and had a film of diesel fuel across it as well as what was probably the waste water from the fully loaded dive boats. We'll hang out another day and then continue on to Sri Lanka.

JANUARY 15, 2006: EN ROUTE TO SRI LANKA

Snorkeling yesterday was great. The water did clear up and the visibility was close to one hundred feet right under the boat. In the shallower water, we spotted a few big green eels and a turtle that didn't mind us following him around.

This morning we left for Sri Lanka and had what turned out to be our best day of sailing in at least 5000 miles. We didn't make great time, averaging only about four knots, but the wind was nice and steady. It was absolutely perfect for throwing out the screecher sail and relaxing.

We had a pod of dolphins join us in the afternoon. There were about fifty swimming all over each other in our bow waves. Eventually they peeled off, but three of them stuck around for close to an hour.

At one point there was a noticeable change to the water. The water we were in was choppy, as if there was a current opposing the direction of the waves, but up ahead

I could see a clear distinction where the water went completely flat. Just as we sailed into the flat water one of the dolphins jumped out of the water and smacked his tail to make a big splash. Kind of weird.

JANUARY 16, 2006: EN ROUTE TO SRI LANKA

There are some strange things going on in these Indian Ocean waters. Throughout the day it went from choppy to glassy in an instant. We see that occasionally, but here it seemed to be every fifteen minutes.

Last night while I was on watch, we were motorsailing in calm seas and light winds. Then suddenly the boat started slamming and bouncing up and down. I raced outside and found the boat bashing through big white cap rolling waves. Our speed dropped to just one knot, which clearly showed that there was a strong current running up against us with the wind causing the standing waves.

I kept an eye on the depth finder though since it felt like some uncharted island was about to rear up from underneath us. Five minutes later our speed was back up to normal and the seas were flat again. It was just long enough to get my heart pounding and to wake Ali from a fitful sleep.

JANUARY 18, 2006: EN ROUTE TO SRI LANKA

This passage has certainly been living up to the hype, becoming our most pleasant ever. We left three days ago, put out the screecher sail and haven't touched it since. With a steady ten-knot breeze, we manage hundred mile days without seeing a whitecap on the water. The forecast for the next four days looks exactly the same. It'll be great if it holds up.

Here is something quirky that we have heard from nearly every long-range cruiser that we have met. After introductions and exchanging pleasantries, about the third question in the conversation goes like this, "So how long have you been out?"

We tell them two years. To which their response every single time is, "Oh, you guys are hurrying."

Then it's, "Yeah, me and Bobbi Jean have been in Thailand for three years now."

Or, "We spent five years in the South Pacific."

Then usually a little later in the conversation they'll let slip that they fly home for six months out of the year to visit the grandkids and go to work.

Our goal is to sail around the world, not to live the rest of our lives on a boat. If that is their dream, great, but it isn't ours. Long-distance cruisers are a strange bunch. It always feels like a competition with them. I don't think Ali and I will ever fit in with this group. In fact we find ourselves avoiding interactions with them more often than not lately.

JANUARY 20, 2006: EN ROUTE TO SRI LANKA

Nothing has changed out here in four days, and for once that is a very good thing. We're still only averaging about one hundred miles a day, but are happy with that since the wind has been so perfect, the temperature ideal, and the skies blue and sunny. We are as tan as we have ever been and are a dermatologist's worst nightmare. We've only had to touch the sail once and that was to roll it up for about a three hour lull when the wind disappeared.

Yesterday at sunset we were sitting outside jabbering away, when Ali looked over my shoulder and jumped up. We didn't even notice a ship had appeared less than a mile away, headed straight across our path. I don't normally radio these ships, figuring they've got better things to do than talk to every sailboat that they go by, but this time I hadn't been watching long enough to know his path or speed.

I gave him a call on the VHF and he came right back saying he would be passing six tenths of a mile in front of us. No problem, but at night that would have scared the heck out of us. It is truly amazing how fast ships can appear from over the horizon. This was the only ship in four days and we crossed paths within half a mile of each other. Sometimes the ocean doesn't feel so big.

JANUARY 22, 2006: EN ROUTE TO SRI LANKA
Still truckin' along. Last night the wind piped up to twenty knots, which is the strongest we've had on this passage. That's a little high for our light wind sail; but since the forecast didn't show any strong winds, we just rode it out through the night. This morning the wind did die down, although it felt like it could come on strong again at any time. We decided that maybe after a full week it was finally time to roll up the screecher and raise the mainsail.

It seems unbelievable, but this is the first time we have raised our main in over three thousand miles. The last time we had the sailbag open was on our sail to the Wessell Islands on the top end of Australia. After that we had the passage to Bali in which we were practically becalmed the entire 1100 miles. Then we had the 1200 mile passage up to Malaysia where we went from being becalmed for days on end to having strong headwinds in which we just motorsailed with the jib.

Granted, a "real sailor" would have raised the main during a lot of that and done some tacking. But tacking is my nemesis, I love to stay on my rhumb line.

From Malaysia we had the quick hop over to Thailand, where again we motored and motorsailed. Then from Thailand we sailed 700 miles with the screecher until this morning when we finally gave in. We weren't sure what to expect when we raised the main. We were half expecting bird nests to fall out of it, but it was clean and looked good. With the wind around twenty knots, it turned out to be the right choice.

We're getting anxious for landfall. Our conversations have been revolving around food, which is always a sure sign that we are ready to get off of the boat. We're not sure what we are going to find upon arriving in Galle. Hopefully there are still a couple of floating docks in the harbor, but with the damage from the tsunami last year we aren't sure if they will be there or not.

JANUARY 23, 2006: EN ROUTE TO SRI LANKA
Only eighty miles to go and I haven't been this excited about a landfall in a long time. I'm not really sure why though. Maybe it's the excitement of the unknown, of not having any idea of what to expect. I mean, I don't know a single person who's ever been to Sri Lanka.

The sailing the last couple of days has been fast, with winds around twenty knots and following seas. Our good mileage has us arriving a day earlier than anticipated, something that never happens. Today we had a few ships cruise by and even a small fishing boat, the first signs of life in awhile. For some reason, despite all the fishing boats, we haven't managed to catch anything ourselves.

JANUARY 25, 2006: GALLE, SRI LANKA

After one of our most successful passages to date, we arrived in Sri Lanka. Ali woke me up this morning as we were being surrounded by fishing boats. I came outside and there were two large boats on either side of us with a half dozen men on each.

They were all happily waving and a few were yelling hello. Then they started making the international sign for, do you have cigarettes? Wanting to trade the fish they were holding up for some. Unfortunately the last thing in the world we need upon arriving at a new place full of restaurants is fresh fish, so we politely waved them off and they turned and headed for home.

We motored along the coast for the rest of the morning. The south coast of Sri Lanka is almost one continuous beach, occasionally broken into different bays by an outcropping of rock. Just before noon we came around the corner and entered Galle Harbor. We could see a few masts sticking up from behind the breakwater and headed in that direction.

At the entrance we were approached by a small boat with two guys wearing uniforms. They told us to stop and informed us we could not enter the harbor. They spoke some English and eventually we figured out that we had to contact an agent, who would send the proper authorities out to the boat.

Our conversation with the agent was hilarious. We knew he was speaking English but could not understand a word he was saying. Ali and I would concentrate as hard as we could while he was speaking, and as soon as he finished we would look at each other hoping that one of us had understood something. Then inevitably I would have to ask him to repeat, to which he would simply speak louder and say it again in the same unintelligible voice. It took us a long time to get through his list of questions.

About an hour later, two nice guys from the Navy poked around the boat a little bit. Then together we motored into the harbor. The dock here is actually just a narrow floating plastic pontoon about a hundred feet long. There is room for ten boats, we were number nine and got stuck on the inside closest to the rocks.

After the Navy left we met our agent. He was a nice man who made repeated comments about my wonderful t-shirt. A none too subtle hint that he would like a t-shirt from us. We ignored it for now and got him to carry on with his work. Soon the agent and I set off for the office to fill out more paperwork.

He had a rickety one-speed bike which he told me to hop on. By that he meant for me to sit sideways on the bar between the seat and the handlebars. We made quite the sight, a frail old man pedaling an ancient rusty bike with a big white guy twice his size balancing precariously between his legs.

This was my first chance to see some of the devastation from the tsunami. He pointed out where huge ships had been lifted right up out of the harbor and transplanted into the middle of the nearby neighborhood. The neighborhood was now gone, only a handful of concrete shells remaining. One large boat was still sitting next to the agent's water-stained office five hundred yards away from the water.

The paperwork was simple, and only the process of making multiple copies by hand managed to slow us down. It took a few hours to complete everything, but by dinner time we had finished up and had our shore passes to prove it.

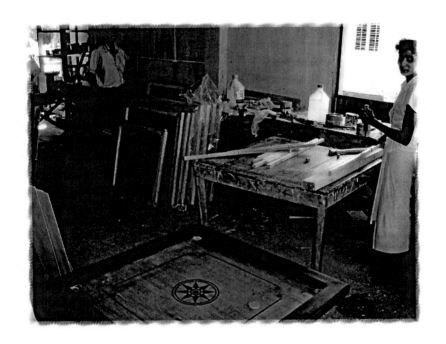

rolled with it

OVER THE NEXT FEW WEEKS Ali and I settled in to life on the island and fell in love with the people. Everywhere we went we were greeted with huge smiles and gracious welcomes. Americans had been among the first to show up in Sri Lanka after the tsunami and it was clear that they had done a lot of good. Person after person stopped us on the streets to ask us where we were from and to tell us a story. The most common was about the day the U.S. Navy arrived. Their eyes lit up as they explained how these giant boats came to shore and then proceeded to drive right up onto land. Amphibious vehicles were quite a novelty.

Every tuk-tuk in the area was new, and had been donated by one country or another. Each driver proudly displayed the country that had made the contribution that allowed him to continue to work. We traveled the island from one end to the other in these tuk-tuks listening to the driver's stories of heartbreak. Everybody had lost somebody close to them.

We spent a lot of time off the boat during our stay. The harbor was a safe place to leave her, as it was protected twenty-four hours a day by the Navy thanks to the civil war raging for the past thirty years. Most of the fighting was centered in the north, but there were the occasional surges throughout the rest of the country. Nothing increases the feeling of safety like a war.

The beaches ran nonstop around the island and we spent time surfing quite a few of them. The breaks were uncrowded, the beaches were scattered with cheap hotels, and the food was terrible. Oh well, it can't all be perfect.

THE WEEKS PASSED QUICKLY, but despite running a bit late in the sailing season we just couldn't bring ourselves to leave. It seemed that every day something great happened. Our revelation in Thailand was already paying dividends. Never before in our lives had we met people who were so open and honest. All we had to do was walk down any road to experience it.

FEBRUARY 6, 2006: MIDIGAMA, SRI LANKA
We decided to take a walk back to the nearest town which we had thought couldn't be more than a mile away. We severely underestimated the distance, but kept going anyway.

At one point we walked by an old lady with three young girls, who were wandering around an empty lot where a house must have stood a year earlier. The old lady waved us over and they all seemed delighted when we did. She spoke fairly good English, but the girls didn't speak any. They seemed to really like Ali and told us how beautiful her laugh was, and marveled at her bright white smile.

The two youngest girls ran off to a nearby shack, which now served as their home, and came rushing back holding two handwoven friendship bracelets. The youngest girl was super shy but managed to tie one of them on my wrist. She was absolutely beaming when she finished and I told her how much I loved it. Ali and I were sort of ashamed for not having a single thing to give to them in return, but not even for a second did it feel like they wanted or were expecting anything.

Continuing down the road, Ali and I couldn't stop talking about how sweet the locals have been to us. As we were walking past a house that obviously had some sort of party going on, an older man stopped us and insisted we join them. We politely declined at first; but he was persistent, and after meeting his nephew, who was about our age, we were persuaded to join them.

They were a family of Buddhists and called the party an alms giving, which was for their grandmother who had died five years earlier. I might not have gotten all the details right, but from what I gathered they go to the temple to worship her and leave food and gifts for her spirit on this day every year. This had all been done earlier in the day and now it was simply a party. There were about thirty people there who all welcomed us before quickly ushering us inside to eat.

We were served up big plates of rice and an assortment of dishes to go with it; fish, chicken, a few curries, vegetables, and on and on. We began to eat like the rest of them, digging in with our hands. But after a couple of minutes the younger group insisted that we eat with a spoon, which was nice since we weren't proving very adept at eating rice with our fingers without making a mess.

Everybody was extremely friendly and we were having a nice time. It felt just like a family reunion back home. The older man who had stopped us on the road turned out to be the uncle of the younger group we got to talking to. After he had asked Ali her name for the twelfth time, they laughingly explained to us that he had been into the *Arrak*. We laughed as well, since it doesn't seem that there is a family anywhere who doesn't have an uncle that hits the sauce a little too hard.

While Ali answered questions about our life in America, I joined in on the cricket match going on out in the yard. I had never swung a cricket bat before so I was pretty excited when I hit the first pitch all the way across the road. Then they told me that wasn't good since apparently if this had been a real match there would have been a guy there who would have caught it. I then tried bowling, but despite being a pretty fair baseball player, they hit everything I threw at them.

Ali continued to be questioned by the girls and had to assure them that we would have children soon. They also asked if I had a brother, because one of the girls was still unmarried at twenty-seven, and they were certain that what she needed was a good American boy to take care of.

We never did get to town that day, but managed to get back to the hotel before sunset. When we pulled up our seats on the beach to watch it, we ordered a couple of beers only to find out that the hotel could no longer serve alcohol. Apparently this was a new government law that was doing an excellent job of lowering both tourist's enjoyment and hotel's profits. So instead of muddling our minds with alcohol we watched a beautiful sunset and called it a night.

FEBRUARY 12, 2006: GALLE, SRI LANKA

Today at the vegetable stand, a nice man who spoke good English started chatting us up. He helped us pick out some good vegetables after grabbing the bad ones that we had chosen right out of our hands. He seemed like a nice guy so we asked him if he knew where we could buy a Carrom board. After playing Carrom, a sort of checkers billiards game at a beach bar one day, I was hooked and wanted one so I could kick Ali's butt every now and then. He told us there was a store nearby that sold them, but that he could take us to the factory which was near the harbor.

He asked us to wait and ran off to fetch a *tuk-tuk*. Ali and I climbed in while our new friend told the driver where to take us. The driver said he didn't know the place, so our friend said he would go with us. Ali and I were starting to feel like we were about to be taken on a ride that would end up costing us a bunch of money, but we had made that pact in Bangkok to try and let our guard down and just see what happens. So once again we just rolled with it and all piled in the *tuk-tuk*.

Just like he said, the factory was on the road right before the harbor. It was actually just a big room, but I guess if you build a lot of just one thing, then you can call yourself a factory. There was a skinny little lady of a completely indeterminate age working on the frame of a Carrom board as we walked up. She seemed quite surprised to see us.

Our friend told her what we were looking for and she invited us to have a look around. We found the board we wanted and after some bargaining we reached a price that everybody seemed happy with. It may have been a little expensive, but we were just happy that we got to buy it direct from this nice lady.

She didn't have the playing pieces though, so our new friend told us he would get them for us and meet us back out front of the harbor in an hour. Before we left I saw the lady give him 60 rupee, the equivalent of sixty cents, which I figured was his cut for bringing us there.

Later on, out front of the harbor entrance with our pieces, we noticed right away that the price on the box was 60 Rp. The money exchanged had simply been to buy the pieces with. Ali and I were headed back to Galle as we had forgotten a few things earlier. Our friend was headed that way too, so the three of us hopped in a *tuk-tuk* and drove back to town. Out front of the bus station we had a nice chat, and we gave him a *Bumfuzzle* baseball cap. He pulled it on happily, we shook hands, and said goodbye as he raced across the street to catch his bus home.

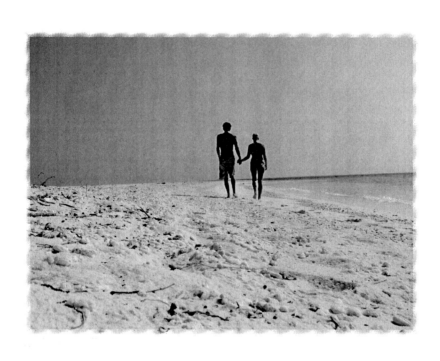

FEBRUARY 14, 2006: EN ROUTE TO MALDIVES

Yesterday morning the Navy arrived right on time. We already had our clearance papers but had to wait for them to board the boat and give us permission to leave. They came on and asked for a crew list. We handed one over and then they asked me to sign it. Everybody then smiled and shook hands, and we were off. I have no idea what receiving a signed crew list was going to do for them, but then again it never ceases to amaze us just how much officials love to accumulate paperwork.

As soon as we pulled out of the harbor, we noticed the big six-foot swell. It seemed to be coming from about three different directions at once and was making things really uncomfortable. We both started popping motion sickness pills, while expecting that once we got clear of land the swell would flatten out. There was no wind so we just motored along bouncing every which way until evening came and the wind filled in.

Throughout the night the wind gradually increased giving us some big seas. We double reefed the main and sailed through the night, with an occasional wave slapping the boat and washing over the top. Fortunately we also had a full moon which makes the rough nights much easier to handle.

At one point I was outside on watch when a particularly big wave slammed into us and woke Ali up. She came outside to make sure everything was okay and I told her that maybe we should put in a reef.

That made her mad since every night before going to bed she runs through a long list of things I have to do while on watch, and one of those things is to wake her up as soon as we need to reef. She says the only time we ever reef is when she comes outside to check on things. That's actually true, but I think it is because we both have different tolerances for what we feel is safe. Though she says for her to feel safe enough to sleep she needs to trust that I will wake her up. So anyway, we put the reef in and before she went back to bed I once again, for the hundredth time, promised to wake her if we needed to reef. This time I really meant it.

Before leaving Sri Lanka Ali did some home cooking, whipping up a batch of potato salad to snack on during the passage. I proclaimed it to be the best in all of Sri Lanka, which she didn't take as a compliment, even though I swear it was.

FEBRUARY 16, 2006: EN ROUTE TO MALDIVES

Only a hundred miles to go now before we reach the Maldives. This afternoon the wind has all but disappeared, though thanks to a strong current we are still making four knots.

We have seen quite a few ships on this passage. Most of them have been to our north on a direct heading for the Red Sea; but last night during Ali's watch, she had to maneuver around one. It had all of its lights on but was just sitting out there doing absolutely nothing. Sort of strange.

FEBRUARY 18, 2006: ULIGAN, MALDIVES

After an easy four-day passage, we arrived at the island of Uligan in the Maldives. The island looks very similar to the Tuamotus back in the South Pacific, flat and small with a beach around the outside and the center covered with palms.

The anchorage is pretty deep, at fifty feet, but we found a place amongst the other half dozen sailboats and were quickly situated. I dived in to have a look at the anchor, but surprisingly the water clarity wasn't very good. I had to dive down thirty feet before I could see the bottom. By the time I did that and climbed back on the boat, I found Ali already had a full compliment of island officers onboard. She got us cleared in and we spent the rest of the day just cleaning up around the boat.

FEBRUARY 19, 2006: ULIGAN, MALDIVES

Today we got the, "Oh, you've only been gone two years, you are really hurrying," line again. That one sentence always puts this abrupt awkward end to any conversation we might have been having up to that point.

FEBRUARY 21, 2006: ULIGAN, MALDIVES

Alright, its official, we can't stand cruisers. We know that cruisers are supposed to be this great, super tight-knit group of fun-loving people, and maybe it's not them, it's us. But we've seriously had it with them.

Yes, we have met a handful of them who are really nice people who don't drive us crazy, but today was the final straw for the rest of them. I wrote about this just two days ago. Two days! And yet, while clearing out with customs today, I was talking to another cruiser and had the following conversation.

"So how long have you been out?" This is how these cruisers start this conversation every time. The second they ask this question Ali and I both know exactly what is going to follow. The truth is that they really could not care less how long we've been out. The real reason they ask is that they want to tell us how long *they've* been out.

"Oh we left Florida a little over two years ago now." Pause.

"Wow, you're really hurrying then." Every freaking time. It's like the movie *Groundhog's Day.*

He paused about a tenth of a second before continuing with, "We left in October of '95, spent three years in New Zealand, two in Australia, blah blah blah blah." I broke in to tell him that it sounded like they were going awfully slow, which seemed to confuse him, and pretty much ended the conversation.

Back at the boat I mentioned to Ali that was the second time that guy told us he'd been out sailing for eleven years. But she told me that this was actually a different guy. I have a hard time differentiating between guys with scruffy gray beards. Nothing against beards, but come on, it's just such a sailor cliché.

So within three days we had two separate eleven-year cruisers, who were well into their sixties, tell us that we were hurrying. And then unsolicited, they try to tell us their entire cruising resumé. The next time anybody asks us how long we've been out, I am just going to walk away, right there in the middle of the conversation.

BY THIS POINT ALI AND I had about had it with cruisers. They all seemed to have this attitude that they were really great, and nothing anybody else did compared to them. Then there were the cruisers that spent their days lurking on internet chat rooms and cruising forums. This group was truly amazing, bashing us for everything from our eating habits to our sailing skills.

Somewhere along the line one of them had made a big fuss over the fact that I didn't know how to tie a bowline. A bowline is a knot that is apparently a prerequisite to being able to go sailing. This was proof positive that the two of us had no business being out here on the water with those that had dedicated their lives to the simple task of sailing a boat.

Truly the only people related in any way to sailing that we were enjoying the company of were the people who e-mailed us. We were receiving dozens of e-mails daily from across the globe, the vast majority of them from people who had the dream to sail around the world. By now we knew that this was something that anybody with enough determination could do, and we actively encouraged everyone to make it happen. We just shuddered to think what would happen to those dreams when they began to talk to these other groups of "cruisers" we had found ourselves surrounded by.

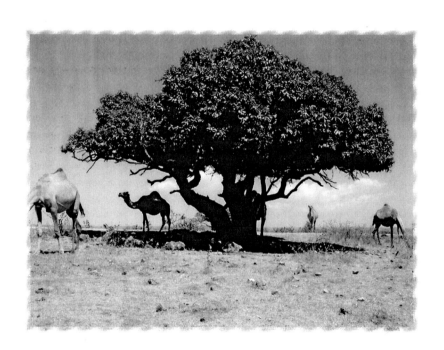

FEBRUARY 24, 2006: EN ROUTE TO OMAN

Already day three of the 1250 mile passage to Oman. Uligan was a nice stop right along our route, and with a string of nearby deserted islands, looked like it would be a great place to spend some time exploring. Unfortunately their rules forbid us from venturing anywhere but the one designated anchorage. With so little to see or do, we quickly moved on.

The first day out, we found ourselves with wind on our nose, but with a little adjusting we were able to motorsail pretty well. By the second day we had caught a favorable current, and now on day three find ourselves flying along at close to seven knots in under ten knots of wind, which is a speed virtually unknown to us.

Otherwise not much going on out here. There have been quite a few ships, which are something we're not used to seeing much of on these long ocean passages, but I suppose it makes sense because anybody heading for SE Asia is coming right out of the Red Sea where we are headed.

We've had the fishing lines out constantly but haven't caught a thing. With absolutely no meat onboard, unless we count the little chunks in a can of chili, we find ourselves dreaming about a big mahi mahi dinner. Amazingly, Uligan, a town of 450, with dirt roads and homes made of coral, didn't have a frozen foods section.

FEBRUARY 26, 2006: EN ROUTE TO OMAN

We are in the midst of yet another extremely uneventful passage. The Arabian Sea has lived up to its reputation as a pretty benign stretch of water. The winds have still been on our nose, keeping us from making very good mileage, but when everything is this calm there's really no reason to complain. The winds are forecast to pick up and shift in a day or so and hopefully we'll get moving a little better then.

Still haven't caught any fish, but we did find some meat on the boat. We've reached a new low here on *Bum*, eating hot dogs from a can. Large pink chemically enhanced hot dogs in a can. We made sure to bury them underneath a can of chili, and without having to look at them, they were pretty good. We really aren't good at grocery shopping for these long passages.

Yesterday was a strange day. There was a sailboat slowly closing in on us throughout the day, which wasn't a big surprise since everybody who was in Uligan, about a dozen boats, would be following the same straight line to Oman. But right as he pulled ahead of us, about one hundred yards up, a big ship came along and passed right next to him. At the same time we had a little Sri Lankan fishing boat pull up alongside of us asking for cigarettes. Three hundred miles from land, and suddenly we had three different boats within a couple hundred yards of us.

We really couldn't believe the Sri Lankan fisherman was out here, nearly eight hundred miles from home. Hard to imagine that they would need to go that far to fish, and then not even offer us a fish to trade. But then again we haven't caught a thing either. By dark the only one left was the sailboat, and by morning even he was gone and we were alone again.

MARCH 2, 2006: EN ROUTE TO OMAN

Only three hundred miles to go to Oman, and there is really nothing going on. We finally caught one small mahi mahi, but somehow managed to lose two others.

About three days ago the wind finally shifted and we had some of that decent sailing weather we had been anticipating. It blew over twenty knots and was from just far enough off the nose for us to sail. It was nice to be sailing, though it was a little uncomfortable since bashing into the wind and waves isn't exactly our best point of sail.

MARCH 3, 2006: EN ROUTE TO OMAN

The wind completely disappeared today, leaving us once again motoring across a motionless pond. Before we set out on this trip, we had no idea that the oceans could ever be so calm. When we are on land looking out at the water, it always seems to be doing something. But out here, on pretty much every passage, including the Tasman Sea, there has been at least one day of seas so calm we could stare at our reflection in the water and fix our hair. On days like this when we are sitting inside, it is easy to forget that we are even moving.

A group of bottlenose dolphins cruised past a little while ago. It's cool to see the big bottlenose dolphins as opposed to the little common dolphins we see most of the time. For the first time we had the big guys doing huge jumps for us.

This afternoon I fixed a couple of blocks, which are the little wheels that our lines run through. They were so sun damaged that the plastic had hardened and begun to crumble. I needed more blocks than we had, so I just switched a couple of them around. On our mast there are four lines running through these blocks. Two are reefing lines and are the ones that needed replacing. One is the main halyard, and then there is the mystery line.

Ali found out what I was doing and sarcastically said, "Oh I'm sure everybody has at least one line on their boat that they don't know the purpose of." And so it is with us, we have this yellow line that runs from the cockpit, through the blocks, into the end of the boom nearest the mast, then along the inside of the boom to the end where it is tied off in a knot. Two and a half years and we don't have the slightest clue why it is there.

MARCH 4, 2006: EN ROUTE TO OMAN

Last night was so dark and calm that the only thing we could see outside were the reflections of the stars on the water. It was the kind of night we both love.

I was sound asleep when I felt the boat lurch up and shudder. It woke me up from a deep sleep so it must have been a pretty big jolt. I remember thinking for a split second that the wind must have really picked up for us to be slamming through waves again. Then Ali, who had been busy making tea, burst in and told me that we had hit something. Within seconds we were on deck peering into the darkness trying to see what it had been.

I've probably read a dozen stories about people running into whales while sailing this stretch of water, so I might just have that bias in my mind making me think that is what we hit, but we're both pretty sure that's what it was. The Indian Ocean is teeming with whales, which sleep on the surface to breathe.

The impact had been on the starboard side only and there was no real noise from it other than a shuddering of the boat as we lifted up. When we hit something hard, like a buoy, it is loud and obvious. The other main obstacle in the oceans are shipping containers that come loose from ships in storms. We've never seen any, but again we've always read stories about them. It definitely wasn't anything like that though. So the only thing we can reasonably assume is that we hit a whale, and fortunately not very hard, since it seems that whatever we hit was rather soft and only glanced off the hull.

It was sort of spooky watching the depth sounder. It stops giving a reading after it gets too deep, but immediately after the impact it read a few feet deep and then dropped down to around twenty-five. For the next twenty seconds it rose and fell between twenty-two and twenty-eight feet before it couldn't get a reading again and just started to blink.

MARCH 6, 2006: SALALAH, OMAN

We arrived in Salalah yesterday afternoon after three solid days of motoring. The land as we approached was a haze of dusty brown, with strips of low white buildings lining the coast for miles.

The harbor is a main shipping port and is filled with huge cranes loading and unloading containers. There is one small section that is set aside for yachts to anchor. With yachts only arriving during a three-month period throughout the year, they don't exactly go out of their way for us, but it's not too bad. The harbor, like in Sri Lanka, is set inside a military compound which makes the running of things much like you would expect a military bureaucracy to be run.

Upon our arrival we called harbor control for details on clearing in. They asked us to standby while they contacted customs and immigration. But while waiting we overheard other yachties on the VHF who all seemed to be having a terrible time trying to clear in. I decided not to wait around all day for harbor control to call us back and instead just headed to shore to contact immigration myself.

The office was nearby, and inside I found a couple of cruisers talking with the one officer on duty. I sat down to wait my turn and could tell it was going to be awhile. And indeed it did take a long time. A couple of hours in fact. But eventually I had the paperwork we needed and we were free to roam about the country.

Back outside I got to talking with a guy from the Coast Guard who spoke pretty good English. He informed me that the reason there was so much confusion was that, "George Bush makes it very complicated for us." He said it totally straight faced, as if my President had personally dictated how this little one man immigration office in Salalah had to fill out paperwork clearing in foreign yachts from around the world.

MARCH 10, 2006: SALALAH, OMAN

The other day we caught a ride into the city and began wandering around. We quickly found that Salalah does not lend itself well to walking. The boulevards are giant expanses of simmering blacktop with a city block seemingly stretching for a mile. We eventually found shelter at a small shop selling ink stamps. We had them make us a simple stamp with our boat name and registration number on it.

As we were talking to the shop owner, we also struck a deal to rent his personal car for a few days. At half the price of the agent lurking around the docks it was a steal. For the next few days we did nothing but drive the empty roads around the desert and the nearby mountains enjoying the beautiful scenery and the thousands of camels that stood everywhere we looked.

MARCH 11, 2006: SALALAH, OMAN

Today a cruiser stopped by the boat and said that he hadn't heard us on the net. He wondered if we knew about it. A net is a cruiser thing that most seem to love, but that Ali and I just cannot get ourselves excited about.

It's like a radio call-in show for cruisers. They all listen in on their SSB radios every day at the same time, reporting their position and what conditions are like. Then after everybody is done with that, they have a section of the show where they exchange information about the places they are at. Now I don't want to sound snobby, because I know ninety percent of people out there would enjoy this sort of thing, but we just have no desire to be involved. When we told him that we don't even have our radio microphone plugged in and that we had never been involved in a net before, he just about choked. He honestly could not believe it.

Apparently they've had these nets going on all the way around the world. Somehow I just can't see what there is to like about having to get on the radio every day at a specific time to report our whereabouts to a bunch of strangers. I mean, I sort of understand that maybe having a big group of cruisers calling in to report what sort of weather they are having might be useful to others around them, but honestly the weather we have had for the last 20,000 miles or so hasn't been worth talking about. I already get my own weather forecasts, and despite all my bitching, the weather is simply never that bad.

The other big purpose of these nets is to talk about places before you even get to them. Personally we hate to talk to people about places we are headed to, because we would much rather explore it for ourselves. We don't want to be told where everything is and what is worth doing and what is not. Part of the fun of a new destination is finding diesel, groceries, and whatever else we need.

I guess more than anything though is that we hate feeling like we've joined in a flock of sheep, and that is what it is starting to seem like around here. The thing with circumnavigating is that each year sort of falls into a group because everybody is following the same seasons all around the world. And right now, here in Oman, we are in a bottleneck. We are all funneling our way into the Red Sea and there aren't a whole lot of choices as far as destinations go, so we start to see each other over and over again. When this happens you get that herd mentality thing going, and we just can't stand it. But hey, I'm ranting for no reason. Some people need that security and that's just fine, what do we care?

ON THE SAME SUBJECT OF GROUP MENTALITY, six boats left the harbor together today. This of course is because we are now heading through pirate waters. Really the only true pirated waters in the world. This is about the only place where there have been attacks against small boats. There is a twenty-four hour period in which we will be sailing through an area that boats get attacked every year. Most cruisers will sail in groups through this area.

Somehow we just can't see the logic in that. If I'm a pirate and I see a group of three sailboats, all I think is that I am going to make three times more money than usual. I just can't imagine why three, or four, or five, or six sailboats together would scare away a speedboat full of pirates. It would be one thing if all cruisers carried weapons. Attacking three sailboats that were all shooting at you would seem pretty stupid, but hardly anybody is packing heat out here and the pirates know that from experience.

So, say for example that Ali and I were traveling in a group of three sailboats and a pirate boat attacks one of the others. What are we supposed to do about it? We have no gun, so we can't shoot them, and our boat is made of fiberglass, so we can't ram them. The only thing I would want to do is run for it, say good luck to our friends and get the hell out of there as fast as we could while the pirates were busy.

At least that is what we would want to do. In truth we would end up trying to go to their rescue, getting robbed ourselves for our troubles. No thanks. We're going to make the passage through pirate territory on our own. We don't need to be worrying about anybody but ourselves.

Honestly though, we aren't worried at all about pirates. According to the numbers I've seen, the odds of being attacked are roughly one in a hundred. In my line of work, if somebody gave me a ninety-nine percent chance of success on a trade, I would lay down everything I owned on it. So why would this be any different? Anyway, we wanted to get that on the record now since it sounds a little hollow if we talk big once we are safely on the other side. Pirates shmirates.

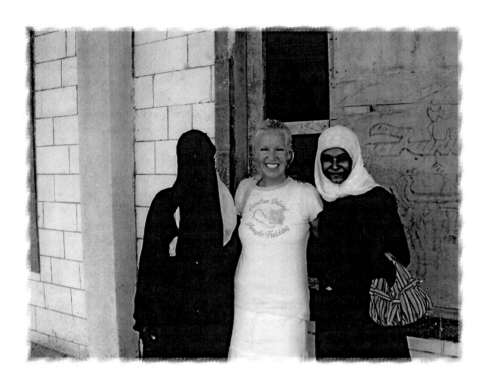

MARCH 13, 2006: EN ROUTE TO YEMEN

Without going into details, we got the, "Oh, you're really hurrying," speech again. This time it was from a younger couple who have taken like ten years to get this far, and have spent at least six years of that back home working. It must be some sort of gag reflex for people to say that to us.

This morning we were on our way out of Salalah at seven sharp. There is hardly a breath of wind, and we are motoring along in calm seas. As soon as we were far enough out we fired up the watermaker. For some reason the watermaker never starts on the first try. This time it didn't start three times in a row, and I began to get really nervous. I messed around with a few valves until eventually it fired up.

Ali didn't seem the least bit perplexed by this whole episode, but for me making water is one of the most stressful times on the boat. I sit there staring at the display, holding my breath, and willing the little green light to appear instead of the red light and blaring alarm. It drives me crazy.

MARCH 15, 2006: EN ROUTE TO YEMEN

Forty-eight hours into another windless passage, and we haven't had a sail up or the engines off. We are supposed to have a pretty strong current in our favor, but so far have been battling against one instead.

Confused by this I have actually put my mask on and stuck my head under the boat to make sure we hadn't snagged a net or anything. Not once, but twice. No nets, but I did jump up the second time when I stuck my head right into the middle of a school of fish. Four little six inch purple and blue striped fish looking as happy as could be were hustling along right underneath the boat. They scooted away for a second when I first stuck my head in but then quickly recovered and continued along just inches from my face.

Yesterday morning we were caught by a convoy. Four sailboats had left in a group just a few hours behind us. One of them had three young boys who were acting pretty funny about this whole pirate business.

They motored a mile out of their way to see us. As they got closer I could see the two older boys running around at the front of the boat, then there was a big bang. They were lighting off fireworks to sound like gunfire, while pointing toy guns and bow and arrows at us. They found the whole idea of pirates to be just another adventure and thought it was pretty hilarious when Ali and I would pretend to be hit by them.

SO FAR OUT HERE we have had two boats approach us. The first was obviously a fishing boat and they did the usual thing, pulling alongside and asking for smokes. The next boat was more of a small open fishing boat that we usually see nearer to land, but this one had two forty-horse outboards and came roaring up to us very quickly.

We could only see two guys at first, but as they got closer two more popped up. We were fifty miles from land so they seemed a little out of place, and I found myself tucking a knife into the back of my shorts. They screamed up alongside of us, looking pretty menacing, but again they turned out to be harmless and just wanted cigarettes.

We went through the usual charade that has to be played out. They make the signal for smoking, we shake our heads no, they repeat, we repeat. We do this between ten and twenty times before they finally take off empty handed. They never ask to trade anything, which baffles me since they are supposedly out here fishing.

MARCH 16, 2006: EN ROUTE TO YEMEN

Yesterday morning I was on the computer when Ali called down to me that we had a boat racing towards us. I quickly changed into some shorts, figuring that I wouldn't cut a very imposing figure wearing boxer shorts, my usual attire while on passage in the tropics.

As always, there was a guy standing at the bow of the boat coming towards us making all sorts of crazy arm gestures. You know how Americans and Europeans use hand signals that we assume are universal? They aren't. These guys have dramatic gestures that we can't comprehend the meaning of. It seems like they are telling us to drop our sails and stop the boat, but we're pretty sure that's not really it.

In any event this group looked pretty rough. I found myself tucking my knife in my shorts again, as if I am some sort of ninja or something. Two of them had scarves wrapped around their faces so only their eyes showed, and the way they were looking at the boat I thought they might seriously be thinking about jumping aboard. But after a few tense moments eyeing each other up they began making gestures that I could understand, begging for cigarettes. After telling them no a few times they roared off. After all of that hype they turned out to be just another boatload of cigarette pirates.

A few minutes later, we were surrounded by similar boats all the way across the horizon. We could see at least twenty of them at one time. They were all coming from the Yemen side of us and heading in the direction of Somalia. The Gulf of Aden is about 175 miles wide at this point and these guys definitely were not fishing boats. We're not really sure what they were all up to. Only the one boat stopped though, and within ten minutes the horizon was clear again.

In the afternoon we had a huge pod of pilot whales join us. This is the first time we have seen these guys. They look to be about three times bigger than a bottlenose dolphin, with a big round head shaped like a torpedo. After about an hour of swimming alongside of us they veered off and disappeared leaving us alone once again.

We're getting into the actual pirate territory now. There is one particular stretch of water, about 150 miles long, where the majority of attacks have taken place in the past. We're running with no lights on at night, relying on the radar to keep us from running into anything. However we do have a full moon which pretty well lights up everything anyway.

So far we haven't picked up anything on radar that we haven't also been able to see running lights on. You have to figure that pirates aren't cruising around with their running lights on, right?

MARCH 19, 2006: ADEN, YEMEN

The last couple of days we transited the area of the Gulf of Aden that is reportedly teeming with pirates. We hardly saw a ship, much less a small boat carrying pirates. There go my dreams of becoming a pirate slaying hero. I suppose it's for the best. Ali doesn't need to be dealing with my ego after that.

We did get a little wind and were able to motorsail, which got us through the area quickly. During the day we were sitting outside keeping an eye on things, when I found myself always looking behind us for boats, and not really paying much attention to what was in front of us. Why did I think that a pirate boat would come up behind us? It's not like we're on a one-lane highway.

THIS MORNING WE PULLED INTO YEMEN. It was the first time in a month that we had overcast skies, which was disappointing since the view was spectacular. Jagged mountains guarded the harbor, with small homes dotting their faces.

As we got closer the water took on that particular shade of green that is used in cartoons to depict radioactive waste. And that's not an exaggeration. This was not a place to go for a swim unless you were hoping to gain some sort of new super powers.

Coming around the corner into the harbor, we were shocked to find about twenty sailboats at anchor. Turns out they were part of a north to south rally. We hadn't really been expecting to find many cruisers.

We dropped the anchor and I put my now fully functional dinghy in the water. My latest super glue patch jobs are doing the trick. I went ashore to get us cleared in and was immediately welcomed by a half-dozen people lingering near the dinghy dock.

I made my way over to immigration and was greeted warmly there as well. We sat down and began the paperwork, which was surprisingly short and sweet. Our new ships stamp, bought in Oman, was a resounding success and was passed around so everybody could inspect it and wonder at where the ink came from. We never did figure that one out.

Next stop was customs, where I was again able to complete the simple paperwork within a couple of minutes. This guy was slick, he asked, "Anything to declare?"

"No, nothing I can think of."

Then in the same tone, and without skipping a beat, he asked, "Any presents for me?"

I patted my pockets and said, "Sorry, nope."

He let it go at that and welcomed me just as everyone else had. Back at the boat, Ali couldn't believe that we were cleared in so quickly.

We were anxious to get off the boat and headed right back in. Walking through town we got a lot of stares and friendly smiles. We were also stopped by quite a few people who asked us where we were from, and then enthusiastically said, "Welcome to our country!"

One old beat up car even backed up a block, going the wrong way, in order to welcome us. It's amazing how much goodwill we have received lately. Back in the States we are made to feel that if we visit these Arab countries we will be attacked by angry mobs. The reality has been quite the opposite.

AS IF TO PROVE MY POINT about not being safer by traveling in a group of sailboats, we met the organizer of the southbound rally while we were at the money changers. We asked how the trip south had gone and he told us that they had lost three boats, out of a group of twenty. Now those are some bad odds. I wonder how many would have been lost had they gone alone.

Two boats hit reefs and were damaged badly enough that they couldn't go on. While another caught fire and sank to the bottom, which it turns out is a very effective way to put a fire out. Don't think the rally organizers will be advertising their success rate on next year's flyers.

Ali tried to cheer the guy up by saying, "Well, at least you've got some exciting stories to tell." He looked at her like she was mad. Apparently he doesn't feel that boat wrecks make very good dinner conversation.

MARCH 20, 2006: ADEN, YEMEN

Yemen has been a total surprise to us. At five o'clock last night we went to the Sailor's Club, a restaurant that we were anchored right out front of. We assumed by the name of the place that it would be another ex-pat hangout, like the Oasis in Oman. But when we walked into the place we couldn't believe our eyes. It was packed full of locals, men and women, drinking and partying.

Every table was stacked high with empty beer cans and bottles of vodka. We sat down and ordered a few ourselves. Pretty soon locals were filing over one at a time, introducing themselves, asking where we were from, and welcoming us warmly to their country.

It was an interesting crowd. One guy was a General in the Yemenese Army who had been schooled in Russia. He had been on the sauce since noon and I soon found myself joining him in a rousing rendition of the Russian national anthem. His girlfriend, a Somalian, was very humorous and was making fun of his drunkenness whenever he had his back turned.

One guy was in Aden visiting his family. He has been living in Detroit for twenty years and insisted on buying his fellow brothers from America a round of drinks. Another girl was from a jungle five hundred miles away near Saudi Arabia. We asked what she was doing in Aden, but she just laughed. Apparently at our naivety, since later on we found out that some, if not all, of the girls were working girls. We didn't know for sure and didn't really care.

I asked our Detroit friend what it was that the locals had tucked in their cheeks. Many of the men had what looked like a baseball in their mouths. The baseball turned out to be a pile of leaves. His eyes lit up as he explained qatt, and the effects of sucking the juice from the leaves. If you use it he said, "Your wife will look like an angel, and the husband will . . ." Let's just say the effects are supposed to be similar to a little blue pill.

Later he appeared with a bag full of these leaves and I popped a few in my mouth. Not that Ali needs any help looking like an angel of course; it just seemed like an interesting cultural experiment. After chewing it awhile I began to feel a lot like a cow. And not a horny cow either, so I threw it out. We went back to the boat soon after. I think Ali wanted to find out if the *qatt* had any effects besides making me look silly.

MARCH 22, 2006: ADEN, YEMEN

All over Aden, at any time of day, people are out on the streets lounging around or playing games. There are billiard and foosball tables on the sidewalks everywhere. Today as we were walking by a group of guys playing foosball they invited us to play a game. I jumped in with them, though Ali, feeling her foosball skills weren't quite up to snuff, let another guy team up with me. We promptly got schooled ten to three. I could blame it on not knowing the table roll, but actually they were just really good players.

MARCH 23, 2006: ADEN, YEMEN

At the dock today we were approached by a group of teenage girls. One of them was really outgoing and asked if she could take a picture with Ali. The girl was really cute and kept telling us, "This is my dream." We couldn't figure out exactly what her dream was, but it seemed just meeting Americans really made her day.

She was one of the more daring young girls we had seen, wearing a standard black robe, but dressing it up with pink cowboy boots, a big pink ring, a pink purse, and taking digital pictures with her pink cell phone. She must have thought she'd met her long lost sister in Ali who was also dressed in head-to-toe pink. After a quick picture with Ali we all said goodbye. But a few minutes later they were back, this time wanting me in the picture as well. It was really a cool experience, and something totally unexpected.

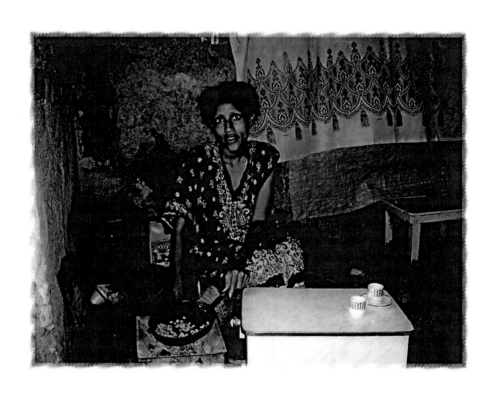

we weren't feeling it

We made it to Africa! A new continent to explore and yet we still haven't stepped foot on land.

Two days ago we left Aden early in the morning for an overnight passage to Assab, Eritrea. This passage took us through the Bab el Mandeb Strait, a ten-mile long pass that leads from the Gulf of Aden into the Red Sea. Throughout the day the winds gradually increased, which we expected since this area acts like a funnel. At midnight we reached the small strait which is only about a mile wide. By this time, winds were up to thirty-five knots coming from behind. We were flying along at ten knots without any problems. It was a little unnerving sailing so quickly through such a narrow area in the dark, but by sunrise we were closing in on Assab and looking forward to a new country.

We tried to hail Assab port control as we approached, but nobody was answering. As we got closer we found the port full of huge cranes and all the normal busy port paraphernalia, except that there was not a person in sight. The wind was still howling, so we just dropped the anchor behind the breakwall and went to bed. By afternoon the wind hadn't let up a bit, and there was no way we were going to put the dinghy in to try negotiating the waves to shore. We decided to just skip Assab completely and continue up the coast without clearing in.

This morning we woke up early and headed out. The winds were still strong, and within a few hours we had seen the first fifty knot winds of our entire trip. Again though, the wind was coming from behind us, and with just the jib out we were sailing along pretty well. Fortunately there isn't enough fetch in this area for the seas to become too big, so despite the high winds the seas never climbed over eight feet.

A little before dark we finally came to our destination for the night, Mersa Dudo. It's a small bay with good protection from the wind, which was still blowing at forty knots when we arrived. After rounding the corner, we had to motor straight into the wind for the last mile, barely making one knot of headway.

Inside the bay we found a fishing boat and a couple of small huts. Before our anchor was in the water, we had a boat full of fisherman motoring over to us. My first thought was that we didn't have enough Cokes in the fridge for everyone. When they came alongside of us, a young kid said hello and then explained that one of the men had an eye problem. He asked if we had any medicine we could give them. Ali and I are not exactly a floating pharmacy, and could only come up with a bottle of Visine. It's always worked on our itchy, scratchy eyes. They thanked us and sped off without another word.

The landscape around here is lunar, exactly what we would expect Mars to look like. Directly in front of us sits a volcanic crater and two giant cones. When the sand haze clears we can see dozens more of these cones in the distance. From the boat we could also see camels wandering around in the black lava flows nearby. Tomorrow we're going to climb a volcano in Eritrea, how cool is that?

MARCH 26, 2006: ERITREA COAST, AFRICA

Today we went ashore to climb the Dudo volcano, but first we walked over to the lava flow where we had seen camels the night before. The area had some greenery, sort of like an oasis but without the pretty little lake they always have in the movies. We thought maybe the camels would be lazing around in the shade but they were nowhere to be seen.

We gave up on the camel search and made our way back across the desert to the volcano. By now our bottle of water had nearly reached a boil and we were slowly roasting as well. It didn't feel that hot out, and the ground wasn't scorching, but the wind carried a steady heat and was still blowing over thirty knots.

The climb up the volcano was pretty easy, just a quick scramble up to the ridge line and follow that to the top. Once there we had a beautiful view of the anchorage, our approach between the islands from the day before, and more volcanic cones as far as we could see. We could also see a goat herder with his flock slowly making their way across the arid ground.

We continued around the crater and then made our way back down to the dinghy. There we found the group of fishermen we had met the day before. They were busy cleaning the fishing net that they had left out to dry on the beach. The kid that had asked us for the Visine came over and told us that the man with the bad eye would like to give us a fish. It was a nice gesture, and we were happy that we were able to help even in such a small way. It can't be an easy life out here.

MARCH 30, 2006: MASSAWA, ERITREA

After two nights at the volcano anchorage, we woke at three a.m. to take advantage of the strong south winds and continue north. Our next stop was far away and we needed the early start. Within a couple of hours the wind had died down and we spent the rest of the day with a gentle breeze from behind.

We reached our intended anchorage an hour before dark but decided to continue on through the night in the hope that if conditions remained the same we could reach Massawa, our next stop, by the same time tomorrow.

We glided past the anchorage as darkness fell. With no moon and overcast skies we couldn't see ten feet in front of the boat. Ali went to bed while I grabbed the iPod and sat down outside to stay awake. As the first song was playing I watched the wind suddenly drop from fifteen knots to five to zero in the space of a few seconds. Something was up.

It then spun around right on our nose and just as quickly climbed from zero to ten to twenty knots. Ali heard the sails flapping and came up to help me drop them while we tried to figure out what was happening. We motored on for about half an hour hoping things would die down again. When they didn't, we decided to head back to the anchorage we had passed by earlier.

After looking over the chart, we found a different anchorage that seemed to have an easier approach and adequate protection from the wind. We would still have to weave through a couple of small islands and their corresponding reefs, but that seemed preferable to getting beat up by headwinds. While Ali watched the charts, I kept a close eye on the radar and depth sounder. We made it in without incident and dropped the anchor.

The next morning we realized why the cruising guide hadn't listed this as an anchorage. The fringing reef that we had thought would be protecting us didn't actually exist and we were pretty much anchored in the middle of nowhere. In the light of day we moved ourselves to a slightly more protected spot.

We went to bed that night not sure if we would be leaving really early again to finish the trip to Massawa, or if we'd sleep in and go to an anchorage at the halfway point. I woke up at two a.m. and found it was completely calm. I never wake up at night, especially in those conditions, so I took it as a sign to get moving again. Because of the Red Sea's predominantly north wind, when we get south winds or no wind we really need to take advantage of it and keep going. The light winds held for us throughout the day and we made it to Massawa by early afternoon.

ERITREA IS AN INTERESTING PLACE. It was an Italian colony until they found themselves on the losing side of WWII and the British took over. In 1952, the Brits handed it over to Ethiopia. The Eritreans didn't like that too much and in 1962 declared themselves a unitary state, touching off nearly forty years of war between themselves and Ethiopia. Looking at a map, Eritrea completely cuts Ethiopia off from the sea, making it obvious why the Ethiopians would want to fight for it. A lot of the fighting was centered around the port of Massawa since it is the largest natural deep water port on the Red Sea.

As we came in we could see the evidence of the fighting everywhere. The port is riddled with sunken ships that we had to maneuver around, and the buildings ashore are largely bombed out shells. The governor's palace has a big dome on top that is half missing and balancing precariously on top of the crumbling building.

We got ourselves anchored and then I headed ashore to get us cleared in. The immigration building looked like it could come down at any moment, but I climbed the stairs anyway and had a seat in their office. While they were filling out the paperwork I had a look around the walls. There were bar graphs all over them. The type you would see in an elementary school, drawn in bright colors on construction paper. There was one for every year listing the number of cargo ships, fishing vessels, and tourist yachts that had called in at Massawa.

In 2004, there were sixty yachts, a couple of dozen fishing boats, and twenty cargo ships. It seemed pretty amazing that a war was fought largely over a port that was handling a whopping twenty ships a year. Eritrea has the second lowest GDP in the world, so I suppose it makes sense that they wouldn't see a lot of cargo ships. There doesn't seem to be a whole lot to trade.

Once cleared in we quickly headed into town to try and find some food and drink. It wasn't hard to find. There were a lot of small local restaurants that were busy putting out tables and chairs and getting set up for the night. We ended up stopping at a restaurant on the second floor of a hotel overlooking the harbor. They served slightly chilled Asmara beer, a nice brew whipped up in Eritrea's capital city of the same name, and handed us menus consisting entirely of the local cuisine, Italian food.

I ordered three things before finally hitting on one that was available, spaghetti. With nothing else on the menu Ali ordered spaghetti as well and we sat back to enjoy the view. We were surprised to find that the locals seemed much more western than we have seen lately. The majority of the women were wearing jeans and t-shirts, with only a very occasional black robe and veil. Everyone was drinking a beer and seemed happy and relaxed.

Walking back to the boat after dinner we saw a line of women sitting in the middle of a dirt parking lot with jerry jugs all around them. We couldn't figure out what they were doing at first but then realized they were all waiting in line to get water out of a dribbling tap. The tap was set so low to the ground that they had to fill a small pail first and transfer that to their jugs. It looked like the sort of thing that they probably spent the better part of a day doing.

There were quite a few restaurants that had filled the streets with tables. As we were walking along I heard Kenny Rogers playing from one. We thought that seemed like a strange choice of music, just like we had thought it was a few months back when they were playing his Greatest Hits in a Kuala Lumpur bar. We were laughing about that when a hundred yards further down the road came a booming, "Lady, I'm your knight in shining armor, and I love you." More Kenny. I wonder if he knows just how popular he really is around the world. We would have liked to stay out for a few beers at one of the local Kenny bars but we were exhausted and called it a night instead.

OVER THE PAST FEW DAYS our boat has become encased in dirt. Our nice white lines are now brown, and the silver mast looks more like a big tree trunk. This is a minor annoyance for somebody like me; but for somebody like Ali, it's a bit more than that. Accordingly, washing the boat has gone from being a once every couple of weeks job, to a daily job. If I wash it off daily with buckets of water, it rinses right away; but if left for much longer, it gets a little too thick and takes some scrubbing as well. Good times.

MARCH 31, 2006: MASSAWA, ERITREA

Yesterday we had a very cool experience. We were walking through town when we came across an old lady who was busy watching a young boy knock a few bricks off of a crumbling building. We said hello as we walked by and she smiled warmly. After a moment she asked if we liked café. We stopped, turned around, and were sort of unsure what she meant. But then she beckoned us to follow her.

She led us to her home and called for her daughter, Almaz, to come from next door. We were welcomed into her home, which, like all buildings in Massawa, seemed to have taken a number of direct hits from bombs, grenades, and machine guns. It was a combination of brick, stone, and concrete, with fifteen foot ceilings, and just one room about fifteen feet square. There was one bed, a small sofa, a couple of plastic chairs, large tapestries hanging on the walls, and a bunch of plastic bags covering the rest of the walls in the areas where it appeared to be crumbling the worst.

Almaz came in moments later with a small metal box that had coals burning on top. She quickly went to work on the extremely drawn out process of making coffee. First she roasted the coffee beans, a ten minute process that filled the room with a delicious aroma. Then she put them in a bowl and ground them. From here the grounds were spooned into a pot, similar to a small genie bottle. She then added water from a plastic container, as there is no running water in the home. The genie bottle then went on the fire. With Almaz constantly fanning the coals the genie bottle sat on the fire for another fifteen minutes. Finally, the coffee was ready.

Already set out were four small espresso-type china cups. Just before pouring the coffee into them she stuffed what looked like grass into the opening of the genie bottle. We asked what the grass was, thinking it was a spice or something, and she told us it was hair from a cow's tail that they used as a filter for the coffee grounds. I don't think that they sell those filters at Wal-Mart.

During all of this, we had been attempting small talk in their limited English and our completely non-existent Tigrinya. We eventually found some common ground that everyone could understand in a photo album from Almaz's wedding. The wedding seemed elaborate and very similar to our own, with a big white wedding gown, a three-tiered cake, and a car decorated with what we assumed said, Just Married on the back. There was even the obligatory picture of the two of them feeding each other wedding cake.

While the coffee was being prepared, we were also given a small shot of gin and a plate of bread with some curry paste. They were obviously eager to share anything they had with us. The bread both looked and tasted exactly like a sponge and was quite disgusting, but we managed a few bites each, which made them happy. All in all it was an amazing encounter in which we got to see exactly what life is like for people here in one of the poorest places in the world. And to top it off, the coffee was excellent.

We also had them exchange some money for us on the black market. They got a nice commission and we got a better exchange rate. When we cleared into Eritrea customs gave us a form in which we were supposed to declare how much foreign currency we were bringing in. We were then supposed to take that form to the bank whenever we exchanged our money for the Eritrean nakfa. Whenever a country forces us to do this we can be absolutely sure that we are getting screwed. The bank rate, as it turned out, was only fifteen to one. The black market rate was eighteen to one. Twenty percent is a pretty major difference, so we were happy to get that done.

We then went to the bank to exchange twenty bucks and satisfy customs. Something that caught our eye at the bank was that there was not a single computer. A bank without a computer seems impossible in our minds, but here they had paperwork stacked to the ceilings.

THIS MORNING WE HEADED INTO immigration to receive our visas. Eritrea would allow us to stay two days without a visa, but if we wanted to stay longer, or travel inland, we needed to shell out the $40 for one. After paying the fee in one office, we had to go to another office to pay seven nakfa each for a manila folder that they put our one sheet of paperwork into before tucking it in their file cabinet. It's sort of funny though, the Eritrean bureaucracy seems pretty involved, but it is actually one of the most efficiently run processes that we've dealt with.

After finishing that, we went back to our coffee friend's home. We had thrown together a little thank you package with some clothes, a picture frame, and a two pound bag of sugar. The picture frame was a hit with mom, and everyone seemed very pleased with the sugar, passing it around in a circle and feeling the weight of it. We're not sure how the shirts went over, but they all had been wearing western style clothes, so we have a feeling we'll see them in a couple of days walking around in their new duds. Of course, they couldn't let us get away with just dropping off our gift, and once again we went through the entire coffee process. They also handed us two eggs on our way out the door. Even Steven.

Later that day, we took a bus over to the next small town of Edaga. The ride cost a mere ten cents. Our intention was to stop in at the long-range bus station and see what time the bus to Asmara left the next day. Instead we found a busy market. We didn't need to buy anything, but watching all the different people was fascinating.

The women wore just about anything. There were a few girls wearing western style jeans and shirts, and a bigger group that wore beautifully colored sarongs in every color and pattern imaginable. There were only a few women walking around in full black gown and veil. The men here are a much rattier bunch, most wearing tattered golf shirts and some sort of khaki pants, or else dressed in camouflage military garb.

We never did make it to the bus station but are certain that there are buses leaving pretty regularly.

APRIL 2, 2006: ASMARA, ERITREA

Yesterday morning we caught a bus to Asmara, the capital of Eritrea, about four hours away. The bus was a small Japanese minibus converted to seat about twenty-five people, a couple of babies, dozens of boxes of salt, possibly some livestock, and whatever else needed transporting.

The first bus we were corralled onto was already full, but they tried to rearrange people, moving them to seats in the center aisle so we could have the window seat. Nobody seemed thrilled with that arrangement, so we backed out and went to the next bus in line allowing us to take our pick of which seat we wanted. Somehow we managed to pick the one with a broken aisle seat, giving us an unprecedented amount of space. We opened the window wide and sat back to enjoy the ride.

As we got underway we were surprised to see everyone start closing up their windows. It was ninety degrees outside, but with the breeze it felt great. Within half a mile all the windows had been shut, except ours. And soon we got a tap on the shoulder asking us to close ours as well. It was crazy.

The second the windows were all closed up the temperature inside the bus soared. We couldn't understand why we were doing this to ourselves. Occasionally a window would be opened for somebody to yell to a friend as we passed by and if it was left open for more than a few seconds people would start to hike up their collars and shiver. The local's body temperature must have been at least forty degrees cooler than ours, because Ali and I were soaked through from the heat.

Besides the temperature the bus ride was pretty nice as far as third-world bus rides go. Our driver actually seemed to care that his bus didn't topple down the mountainside in a ball of flames, which was a pleasant change. Of course he loved his music, and he loved it on full blast. Ali and I are now singing ballads to each other in Arabic. "Ashtaak, ashtaak, ashtaak, w-asaal a'ankoum el-ashwaaa."

The mountains were interesting in that they were tiered every twenty feet. At a distance each mountain appeared to have hundreds of horizontal lines across it, but up close you couldn't really see them at all. I figured at first they were just natural paths, but then noticed that the stones were piled up into nice even walls for miles and miles.

I can't imagine who did all that work, but it seems to keep the mountainside from simply washing down to the bottom when they do get rain.

The locals on the bus were extremely quiet, which is something we are getting used to here in Eritrea. They don't show any interest in us at all, which is fine, but it does feel a little strange after our experiences pretty much everywhere else.

Our bus made one stop along the way for everyone to get off and take a break. Soon a hundred kids surrounded the bus selling little straight sticks that are used as a toothbrush substitute. The locals peel the bark back from one end and mash it up until it looks like a brush, then they sit there all day rubbing their teeth with it.

By the time we reached Asmara, we were filthy and exhausted. We quickly found ourselves a hotel, haggled over the price until we'd reached fifty percent off, showered, and went to bed.

WITH NO SPECIFIC PLANS FOR TODAY we just went out and walked aimlessly around town. The sidewalk cafés only appeared to be for tea and coffee, so for a beer we eventually found ourselves popping in on some of the local bars down the backstreets instead.

Our first stop didn't have much atmosphere, pretty much relying on the thirteen inch television with EriTV blasting at full volume for entertainment. Next door though we found Bar Africa (all the bars have single word names, and all are about as unique as this one) to be much more interesting.

Inside was a billiards table with a bunch of men gathered around in the midst of an intense game. We sat down and watched them play for a while. They called the game billiards, but it was totally different than our billiards back home. It was actually just like bocce ball except on a table instead of a lawn. The locals continued to be extremely quiet with us, until one guy finally gathered up the courage to say hello and tell us a little about the game.

While playing their game everybody kept one eye on the table and one on us. Ali was the only woman in the place, which can sometimes be a little awkward, but when we left she gave the guys a big smile and said goodbye. They all instantly smiled, waved, and yelled goodbye as we walked out the door. Sort of like shy little schoolboys.

Today we realized how much our standards have changed as far as bathrooms go. At Bar Africa I made the scouting mission and came back to Ali with a glowing review. I told her, "It's great! It's just right down at the end of the alley, AND there is even a piece of metal you can use to lock the door." We now tend to overlook the fact that the toilet is just a stinking hole in the middle of a dirt floor.

APRIL 3, 2006: ASMARA, ERITREA

At each bus station there is one guy that seems to run the show. He is in charge of putting people on the buses and determining what can and can't come along. We found this guy and he led us around to an empty bus, putting us in the front row behind the driver. We couldn't be more pleased with his seat choice, because on the bus ride here the other day, the driver and the front seat passenger had been the only ones with their windows cracked. So we figured we'd be getting a hint of a breeze on this trip.

An hour later with the bus now full, we got underway. Ali and I looked at each other and said at the same time, "That was fast." Once again proving just how low our standards have become. An hour wait now seems lightning quick.

The bus pulled onto the main road outside of town where suddenly all of the windows closed at once. The passenger girl left her window open a crack but we weren't feeling it. Our driver completely closed up and then we realized that for some reason our window didn't open at all. We were sealed in again.

A half an hour later the sweat was dripping down our backs and puddling up on the seat. After that came the smell. The smell of thirty people in a metal can crawling down the road under the noon day sun in Africa is something we won't soon forget.

Not too much later we began to hallucinate. Or maybe we weren't, since we all saw the same thing. We were still high up in the mountains when we saw a couple of huge apes with red butts on the side of the road. Then a few more, and a few more, until suddenly a couple of the biggest were screaming and chasing the bus down the road. Maybe angry screaming apes are the reason for the closed up windows.

The next hour passed with the two of us in and out of consciousness before the doors finally swung opened and we stumbled out into the cool eighty-five degree breeze for a quick twenty minute break. There we downed a hot cup of tea, seeing as that is the only beverage available anywhere, and then it was back on the bus to perform an instant replay of the previous two hours. It was torture. The worst part of all was not knowing why in the world these people would do this to themselves. It was beautiful outside for crying out loud.

APRIL 8, 2006: ERITREA COAST, AFRICA

We spent yesterday getting ready to leave again. As usual on our last day in port we stopped to pick up our laundry. Without fail, everywhere around the world there is somebody looking to do cruiser's laundry. I remember before starting this trip we actually contemplated installing a washer on the boat. We didn't go that far, but we did go out and buy two big buckets to do laundry in by hand. Those buckets made it as far as New Zealand before being given away, unused.

Mike, café owner and local dockside go-to guy, helped us out with diesel, black market money exchanging, and the purchase of thirty rolls of bread. With no sliced bread in the country, I wondered to myself what saying they use in place of, "It's the best thing since sliced bread."

We paid Mike what we thought was fair, which wasn't easy to work out in a place where a cup of tea costs four cents. I think maybe we overpaid since he then insisted that we go to his home and have coffee with his family. This despite the fact that we were sitting in Mike's café, which served any kind of coffee we could want from a gourmet machine. Instead we went off with one of his daughters to his home for coffee the old fashioned way, with cow's hair.

We also took the bus over to Edaga again to pick up a few vegetables at the market. We were wandering around buying our stuff when we ran into the old lady who had us to her home for coffee when we first arrived. We stood and chatted for a couple of minutes, and almost felt like a couple of locals just shooting the breeze with our neighbor. Almost.

IN THE AFTERNOON WE DECIDED to press our luck and try to clear out. We knew the official rule was that once cleared out you had to leave immediately. But we figured it was only an hour before quitting time and we'd be gone in the morning before they got to work.

Once we completed all of the formalities, the immigration officer stood up and said, "Okay, let's go out to the boat." We had read about this in our cruising guide but were hoping that this procedure had since been abandoned. He wanted to come out to our boat and check for stowaways. As if there is even a remote possibility of a stowaway being on a cruising sailboat. We hemmed and hawed, eventually giving in and telling him we didn't want to leave until morning.

At seven I was waiting outside the immigration office, and fifteen minutes later our man rolled into work. He gathered his paperwork and together we went off to inspect the boat. He looked around in a state of awe. It's generally pretty uncomfortable having locals on the boat, because in their minds our boat seems so lavish. They invariably ask us how much it cost, to which we make up some ridiculous number like $5,000. In many of these places we could say $500 and it would have the same effect.

It was pretty clear he wasn't looking for stowaways but that the true reason for the visit was for some *baksheesh*. Eventually he got around to asking if we had any water. We poured him a glass and then he asked if we had any extra CDs. "Country music," he hopefully clarified. "Kenny Rogers perhaps?" Ali and I both laughed at that last bit. I might have said no if it hadn't been for his request for Kenny. But the computer was already fired up and I wouldn't be a true American if I didn't have Kenny Rogers' Greatest Hits on there. I burned him an illegal copy, hoping Kenny wouldn't mind the copyright infringement in this instance.

A FEW HOURS LATER than we would have liked, we were underway. We spent all day motoring in very light winds, and are now sitting at anchor in front of an extremely flat, nothing of an island. After anchoring I dove in to check things out and make sure the anchor had set good. Since I was out there, I figured I should scrape the bottom of the boat as well.

The grass that had been growing a little while back had disappeared, with the antifouling paint and a bit of sailing apparently doing the trick. But sitting in Massawa harbor for the last week had been some sort of breeding ground for barnacles. The outside of the hulls, and the props, were completely covered.

Scraping barnacles off isn't hard work, but it is disgusting. Inside the barnacle shells live these bugs that look like miniature crabs. As I scrape, millions of them are released into the water all around me. They can bite a little bit too, making the process even more uncomfortable. By the time I finished scraping the hulls clean, they covered my body, especially enjoying any place with hair. Now, an hour later, I sit here watching as the sun sets behind a true desert island, and write about having crabs in my shorts.

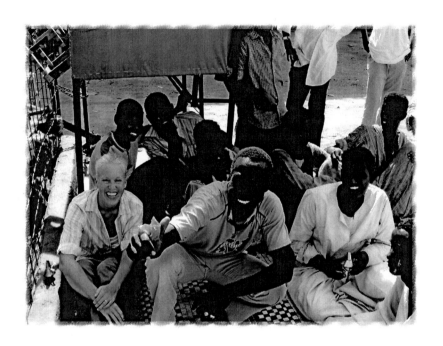

my wife very nice

APRIL 10, 2006: SUDAN COAST, AFRICA

When we went to bed the other night it was nice and calm, but by midnight a south swell had invaded and was making things very loud and uncomfortable. We hardly got any sleep, being woken every five minutes by the noise.

As soon as it was light enough to see, we were preparing to get out of there. We just about had the anchor up when Ali yelled out that there was an exposed coral head only twenty feet in front of us. As the waves washed over it we could see it clearly sticking out of the water. At this point we were directly above our anchor. We finished bringing it in, and quickly backed out towards deeper water. That coral head definitely was not there the night before when I had dove down to check the anchor. We must have dragged in the night. Hitting that in the dark would have been a rude awakening.

We motored throughout the morning until the wind suddenly shifted, allowing us to raise the sails and shut off the engines. It's always a bit surprising when this happens, and even more so in the Red Sea which is renowned for headwinds and nasty weather.

In the afternoon we were closing in on our anchorage for the night, but with the wind at our back we decided to make an overnight run further up the coast to our first stop in Sudan. It turned out to be a good choice as the winds held out for the rest of the day before dying away after dark, allowing us a good night of sleep while motoring.

In the morning the wind picked right back up and we were sailing again. By late afternoon we had covered 200 miles since leaving Massawa and were dropping anchor in a nice little spot along the coast of Sudan.

APRIL 12, 2006: SUDAN COAST, AFRICA

The winds have picked up the last couple of days, so we are still relaxing at anchor in Khor Narawat. Yesterday morning we had a small boat with a machine gun mounted on it, and four guys in passable uniforms, pull up alongside of us. One of them came aboard while the others sat back and watched. He spoke really good English, at least ten sentences worth, and was very pleasant. He took a quick look at our passports and told us we were welcome for as long as we'd like.

Then, since we were now such close friends, we had a quick discussion on why Ali and I didn't have kids yet. That one never gets old. A couple who didn't have kids because they couldn't would probably breakdown in tears five times a week while talking with the locals here in Africa. They are relentless with the question of family.

The soldier and I were shaking hands and saying goodbye when Ali decided to go back inside. He then immediately turned to me and asked if we had any cigarettes or alcohol. Men will not ask for anything as long as Ali is around, but as soon as she's gone they start begging. This guy had been really nice and it was clear from our anchorage that they were a long way from home, so we gave them a couple packs of smokes and told them we didn't drink. Pretty harmless.

Tonight while cooking dinner, Ali told me that I could let our stowaway from Eritrea out any time. Maybe we could put him to work cooking, doing dishes, or washing the boat. Something like that.

APRIL 14, 2006: SUAKIN, SUDAN

We were up at three a.m. yesterday for another day long run to our next anchorage. Leaving a place like this, at three in the morning, wouldn't have been possible ten years ago, but now electronic charts are so exact that we aren't even nervous about navigating through reefs and around numerous islands in the dark.

The Sudanese coast is littered with small islands and reefs, five miles out from land with no navigational markings. In most places around the world, a coastline like this would be nothing but blinking lights after dark to warn the unsuspecting mariner. There must be a ton of sunken ships here.

We took off early and by the afternoon were pulling into Suakin, thirty miles south of Port Sudan. Port Sudan is a major port city of about three million people, which makes the small town of Suakin the easier, less crazy of the two used for clearing into the country. It is also one of the coolest looking places we have ever sailed into.

After winding a couple of miles inland, the waterway splits off and comes to Old Suakin, an ancient port city dating back a couple of thousand years, though it's hard to say just how old the buildings are. The cool thing is that the buildings, or what is left of them, are made of coral. The whole place is crumbling but there are a couple of buildings whose shells are still pretty well intact. To reach the anchorage, we had to motor right in close to shore just a few yards from the edge of these buildings where families were strolling among the ruins and men were fishing along the shoreline.

APRIL 15, 2006: PORT SUDAN, SUDAN

We made our way to the bus station early this morning for the short ride to Port Sudan. The bus was crowded, but was gloriously lined with open windows. These Sudanese know how to ride in style. Along the way the road was packed with camels, goats, donkeys, and beat up Toyota pickup trucks.

The homes and living conditions along the highway through the desert were extremely poor, probably the worst we have ever seen. Most homes were only eight feet square and cobbled together with anything they could find. Other homes seemed to be more for the nomadic goat and camel herders. These were tents, five feet off of the ground, patched together from dozens of miscellaneous scraps of fabric, and held in the air by sticks.

IN PORT SUDAN THE FIRST THING that struck us was how few women there were. Thousands of men roamed the streets but hardly a woman could be seen. We didn't have anything important to do, so we just started wandering aimlessly around town checking things out.

We noticed that the town was divided into distinct districts. There was the garment district where dozens of shop fronts were lined with men sewing robes using antique sewing machines. There was a market full of fruits and vegetables with some of the first English-speaking locals we've come across trying to sell us their stock. Another street was nothing but telecommunications and cell phone outlets. It seems that no matter how poor and run down a place is you can always count on there being plenty of cell phones and satellite dishes.

By eleven it was so hot we could hardly move. That's when we stumbled across an internet café. Air conditioning and high-speed internet, what more could we ask for?

After internet and lunch, we started making our way back to the bus station. Along the way we noticed some teenage kids sitting on a mat having coffee. The coffee pots were boiling over a fire built inside a broken chunk of road, with the mat in the shade of a garbage bin. It was a coffee shop, though not exactly Starbucks. As we walked by they all smiled and asked us to join them.

They were all pretty excited when we sat down with them, and were full of giggles and hellos. The young guy who was running the show quickly served us each a tiny pot of coffee and miniature cup filled to the rim with sugar. We poured ourselves cup after cup and whenever our sugar went under halfway, he would top us off again. We had begun to draw a crowd, and soon there were dozens of people slowing down to watch us, or stopping to say hello and practice a few words of English.

We asked if we could take a picture and they eagerly said yes. After each photo they all clamored around to have a look at themselves. We're always surprised by this since almost all of them have top-of-the-line cell phones with cameras built in. Yet picture taking still remains a novelty.

After the pictures a young boy came up to me, and while pointing at Ali asked, "Your wife?"

I said, "Yes, my wife."

Still pointing, and with a big smile on his face he said, "My wife very nice."

When it was time to go I asked what we owed for the coffee. The young kid running the place wouldn't hear of it, and would not accept a penny. We thanked him, said our goodbyes, and continued down the road, happy that we had stopped and had taken them up on their offer.

It had been a fun day in Port Sudan, a place that has got all those things that we love about cities: vibrant colors, a whole lot of hustle and bustle, and that certain urban stink you cannot find out in the country.

APRIL 18, 2006: SUAKIN, SUDAN

Today we had set aside for exploring Suakin. First up was a wander around the coral ruins of Old Suakin. We walked up to the main entrance and found three guards sitting there bored out of their minds. They produced a book of tickets with a cost to us tourists of five U.S. dollars each. Seeing as that was all the money we had on us, we decided to give it a miss. We can see most of the buildings from our dinghy anyway.

Instead we walked to the bus station and caught a pickup taxi for the two-mile trip up the road to the main market district of Suakin, which is located closer to the main highway than the rest of town. The locals in the back of the truck with us were very friendly, and we were laughing and taking pictures the whole ride in.

The main road through town is lined with one-story buildings selling sandals, cell phones, miscellaneous groceries, and goat heads. Ali was dying to try out her favorite goat head recipe for dinner but we couldn't agree on a fair price. We walked away empty handed, keeping an eye out for a restaurant instead. After walking the length of town, we circled back to a little roadside restaurant for some *ful*, a slow-cooked stew scooped up with flatbread.

There were nearly a dozen pots warming, all with different ingredients. The owner was happy to let us have a peak inside each to pick one out. We found our favorite, a simple bean stew with onions and a couple of other miscellaneous vegetables. Two bowls of *ful*, bread, a couple of Pepsis, and a cup of tea for dessert, all for two bucks. Down the road we stocked up on a couple weeks worth of bread and vegetables, and we still hadn't spent the 2,000 Sudanese dinars we'd exchanged.

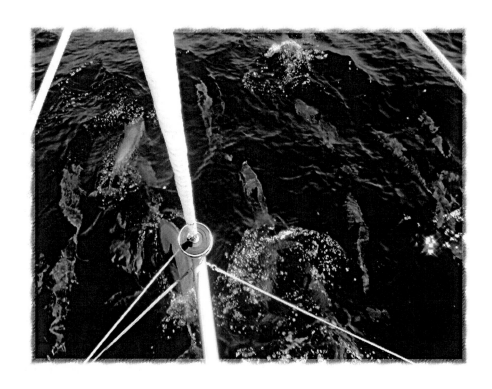

five-minute recess

APRIL 20, 2006: SUDAN COAST, AFRICA

Early this morning we left to make a fifty-mile run north with sunny blue skies, and a light following breeze. Around four o'clock we made our approach to Marsa Fijab, our anchorage for the night.

The entrance here is through a break in the reef which then follows a winding path for about a mile through numerous coral heads. It looked pretty straightforward in the cruising guide, and our charts had good detail, so we weren't at all concerned as we made our way in, despite the fact that the sun was getting low in front of us making the reef harder to see. We followed our now normal procedure, keeping Ali down below on the charts while I steer the boat with one eye on the water and one on the cruising guide.

As we got close to the entrance, something didn't look right when compared to what Ali was telling me was on our charts. I came to the snap decision, wrongly it turns out, that the reason it looked off was that a buoy was missing. In this part of the world, there seemed to only be about half of the number of buoys and channel markers that are shown on the charts.

We continued in and were about fifty yards away from another buoy when I suddenly noticed a distinct change in water color and saw the depth finder climbing rapidly from eighty to fifteen feet. We were already moving slowly, so I jammed us into reverse to stop the boat. As I did so we floated over a coral head at just eight feet. By now Ali was next to me, and we were pouring over the chart in the cruising guide trying to figure out what was wrong.

We finally realized that we were next to a completely different buoy, and that our electronic charts were off by a huge margin, at least a couple of hundred yards. This was the first time, other than a couple of minor details in marina-type areas, that our charts had been incorrect. If the weather had been bad when we tried to come through we could have easily found ourselves in serious trouble. Fortunately we had calm conditions and were able to simply back the boat out the way we had come and slowly creep our way in by sight. No worries.

APRIL 21, 2006: EN ROUTE TO EGYPT

Looking over our weather files the past couple days, we were pleased with what we were seeing. The three-day forecast showed virtually no wind. With 380 miles to go until our clearance port in Egypt, we decided that we'd had enough of the forty-mile day hops and this was the perfect opportunity to make a run for it.

So after blindly fumbling our way out of the Marsa Fijab anchorage we started north. It was another beautiful day and we were motorsailing nicely with just the port engine running. After a few hours we reached what would be the last of our reef areas before we made it out to the deeper water further offshore.

Our charts for the area weren't very detailed, so Ali and I were both out on deck keeping an eye on the reefs, one hundred yards away on either side of us. The water was two hundred feet deep but occasionally would shoot up to fifty, at which point we could see the bottom as clearly as if it were five.

As we stood there we suddenly heard a weird clunk that sounded as if we had hit a small log or buoy. I was standing at the back of the starboard hull watching behind us to see if anything popped up to the surface, but nothing did. I decided to put on my mask and have a quick peek under the boat. I stuck my head in, had a look around, and thought, huh, that's a new one. Our prop was gone. The noise we heard was the prop sliding off the shaft and hitting the rudder before falling down to the ocean floor.

Engines are awfully big and have lots of parts, a couple of which I even have spares for. But there is one spare I don't have that is really, really necessary in order to make the boat go, and that is a prop.

With 350 miles to go, we now have just one engine. What the hell, we needed a little challenge anyway. I don't know if monohullers bring an extra prop along, but I do know that I was once again very happy to have two engines.

To brighten the day we did have a couple groups of dolphins visit us. First came the little guys and then later the big bottlenose.

APRIL 22, 2006: EN ROUTE TO EGYPT

Today we had an adverse current combined with just enough wind on the nose to create small waves and really slow us down, as we plodded along with no sails and one functioning engine. Our speed was under three knots all morning which is really a depressing rate to be moving at.

For some reason our slow speed didn't keep the dolphins from enjoying our company though. We had a huge pod, maybe close to 250 of them, stay with us for hours. We sat up on the trampolines and watched them until the sun became too much and we had to retreat back inside. Eventually the wind shifted slightly and our speed picked up. For a couple of hours anyway. Now in the middle of the night we are motoring along in total calm.

APRIL 23, 2006: EN ROUTE TO EGYPT

I know I talk about them all the time, but they are so cool that I just have to. Today a group of dolphins were floating in a big circle about a hundred yards away from us. There was zero wind, making the water so calm we could watch their fins move lazily across the top. Then all of a sudden it was as if their teacher told them they could have a five-minute recess.

They broke rank and began screaming towards us, jumping over and racing each other. From the top of the boat we could see them perfectly the entire way, even the looks on their faces. They swam with us for a few minutes and then just like that they spun and raced back in the direction they had come.

Despite the fact that we've probably replayed that scene a hundred times on this trip it never becomes any less exciting. It's become almost impossible for us not to personify them. We wonder what they are thinking, if they know that we are standing right above them, if they are trying to impress us, and why they aren't the least bit afraid of a boat that is so much larger and louder than they are.

APRIL 24, 2006: EN ROUTE TO EGYPT

After three days of great sailing/motoring weather, things took a turn for the worse. Yesterday we sailed downwind all afternoon with the screecher in twelve knots of wind. We were amazed since those winds are relatively unheard of in this area of the Red Sea.

Just after dark the wind shifted closer to the nose and then died away completely. At this point we were still pretty happy. We now had flat calm seas and were motoring with a favorable current at over five knots. Then within minutes the wind climbed from zero to twenty knots on the nose. In another hour, it was blowing thirty knots and we were being forced to tack way off course, out towards the middle of the Red Sea.

The forecast had shown nothing over five knots, so we bobbed through the big waves fully expecting that it would pass through. But after pounding away for a few hours, we finally gave up and decided to turn back to the last reasonable anchorage we had passed by earlier in the day.

Normally this is an easy decision for us, but with the loss of one engine we were reluctant to enter an area full of coral. The boat is extremely hard to maneuver using just the one engine; and if we were to get ourselves lost in the middle of a coral field, we could be in serious trouble, especially with thirty knots of wind.

It took us four hours to cover the ten miles back to the anchorage. The last three miles we had to motor directly into the wind and waves with no sails up and just our one tiny engine chugging away. The area we were headed for was called Fury Shoals, a large area of shallow water with a few different reefs dotted around it.

We finally came to our chosen reef; so chosen because it had the least amount of offlying coral heads surrounding it. Inside the horseshoe shaped bay there were a couple of large mooring balls floating right next to the reef. We happily motored up, tied onto a mooring, and settled in to watch the big waves crash against the reef just fifty yards away.

The nice thing about this unexpected stop is that the snorkeling is so good. I went for a swim today and found that I could see the bottom perfectly in eighty feet of water. It's been a long time since we have had that sort of clarity. Along the reef I found the best coral of the entire trip. The colors were amazing, and combined with the white sand on the ocean bottom the entire area just seemed to glow.

APRIL 26, 2006: PORT GHALIB, EGYPT

Yesterday morning we went out for more snorkeling. Not all that many fish, but the coral was really cool the way it shot straight up from eighty feet to just one foot below the surface, and the entire wall was colorful and alive.

After a couple morning swims, we settled down in the afternoon for some beer and cards. While sitting there we began to realize that the boat was shifting and the wind was now coming from the south, perfect for sailing up the coast.

We made the snap decision to get picked up and make the overnight run to Port Ghalib. We were a little nervous a couple hours later as the wind started shifting towards the north. But as it did, it slowly died out, and we spent the rest of the night motoring through calm seas yet again. By afternoon we were safely ensconced in an Egyptian marina.

It's funny, we had a lot of anxiety about this trip up the Red Sea due to its reputation for ferocious headwinds. Something that neither us nor the boat handle very well. Yet in the end the sailing has been nearly as easy as the trade wind belts. I'm now convinced that every sailing book I've ever read has embellished their story to make their journey seem much harder and more heroic than it actually was.

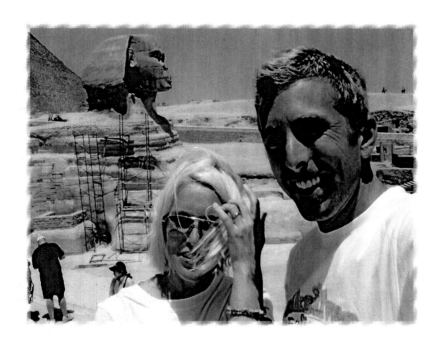

cruising is a competition

APRIL 30, 2006: CAIRO, EGYPT

Port Ghalib is situated in the middle of nowhere, and the marina complex itself was feeling like a prison after just a couple of days. We needed to make an escape, but to do so we needed someone on the inside. We talked to a few marina employees, trying to glean some information on how exactly we could get ourselves out of there and up to Cairo, but we weren't getting anywhere. Not even the resort's travel agent was talking.

The only advice we got was to fly to Cairo on their twice weekly shuttle flight. That sounded terrible. Not to mention expensive. Then finally the hotel manager came through for us. It was like a lightbulb switched on in his head and he suddenly said, "Oh, there is a local bus every night at seven that runs up the coast to Cairo." Perfect!

That night Ali and I stood at a crossroad in the desert and waited for a bus that we weren't entirely sure would even let us on. We were feeling a bit out of place as locals came and went, some sharing a taxi, and some riding in the back of trucks loaded with camels. Eventually one of them approached us and broke the ice, making us feel welcome, and assuring us the bus would be there at seven.

Now nearly an hour late, we were beginning to wonder if the bus would ever show, when it came roaring over the hill. A few locals made a mad dash for the door and we joined in. The driver's assistant jumped off and stood there like he was a bouncer at Studio 57, picking and choosing who would get on. Thankfully he recognized us right away as famous American television actors and let us in.

The bus was much better than we had expected. It was an old tour bus that had gotten a little too shabby for a resort to use anymore but was perfect for the local riff-raff. Ali and I got the last two seats right in the back above the heat of the engine. We were just happy to be on our way to Cairo.

The ride was relatively uneventful and stopped every hour or two for a few minutes of stretching and buying snacks. A couple of very nice twenty something guys sitting in front of us came back from one outing and handed us a whole bunch of junk food. Ali was really excited to see Twinkies again, at which point we realized that our tastes in food haven't changed a whole lot since we were ten years old. Our favorite food was pizza; favorite drink, cherry Kool-Aid; favorite dessert, Hostess snack cakes.

WE HAD BEEN COMPETELY UNSUCCESSFUL in locating a guidebook for Egypt. So when we arrived in Cairo at five a.m. we had no idea of what to do or where to go. It seemed the simplest thing would be to head for a major hotel to get our bearings. We grabbed a cab and took off.

The strange thing about cabs here is that we don't haggle over price before the ride. Instead we are expected to know a fair price in advance and to simply hand it over upon arrival. Of course when we do that there are two reactions. One is a simple nod of the head. What this means is that they are happy because we have grossly overpaid. The second reaction is for them to stare at us and keep motioning with their finger as if we should continue to pile money in their hand until they say stop.

We've found a nice little trick that seems to be working pretty well. What we do is pay as low as we think we can get away with, but also hand over two Marlboro cigarettes with the money. That always gets a smile and seems to help buy us time to get out of the cab without incident. We've taken to carrying around a pack of cigarettes just for situations like this.

As a rough estimate from what we've seen so far, I would say that the number of smokers here is hovering at around ninety-nine percent. Egyptians smoke everywhere. I can't wait to go to the National Museum and see them standing around blowing smoke rings at a three thousand year old mummy.

We arrived at the Nile Hilton and strolled in like we belonged there, heading straight to the café for breakfast, and to kill a couple hours. After lounging around for ninety minutes we began to feel like interlopers, so we relocated to the lobby. It was now all of seven a.m. We were actually waiting for the bookstore in the lobby to open so we could get ourselves a guidebook, but after another half-hour we decided to ask when that would be and found the shop did not open until ten.

We decided to just strike out on our own and search for a hotel. After wandering around aimlessly for an hour we gave up on that idea and caught a cab. I thought I had remembered reading that there was a large bookshop at the University.

The cab took us to Cairo University on the other side of that little river, the Nile. When we got there the guard wouldn't let us through but he told us to wait. He then went in and started stopping students until he found one that spoke English. She came over and was all smiles as she explained that the bookstore here wouldn't have what we needed but that we should go and try the American Cairo University, which as it turned out was only a block away from where we had just been sitting for hours.

After another cab back to where we had started, we found the University bookstore and felt like we were in a Barnes and Noble. The place was huge and had everything. We hadn't seen a proper bookstore since New Zealand and couldn't believe our eyes. We found a guidebook and were finally on our way to a hotel.

THE FIRST HOTEL WE TRIED was a terrible dive, but it was on the same street that the Volvo parts supplier we had tracked down on the internet was on. We were counting on this place having our replacement prop, and quickly headed over there. We walked over and circled the building twice looking for some sort of entrance, but couldn't find one.

There was a Perkins engine shop a block away, so we stopped in there to ask. They didn't know what we were talking about but when we showed them the name and address of the place we wanted, they all got in a huge discussion between themselves.

It's fun to watch one of these boisterous Arab conversations. We can't understand a word of it, but enjoy seeing how animated and loud they get. It seems like there is a heated argument going on, even though it is just a discussion over directions.

After a few minutes the girl who spoke some English wrote the name and street number in Arabic for us and told us it would be easiest to catch a cab. So back in a cab for the fifth time that morning, we figured we would be there in a minute. Half an hour later we were still driving in circles.

Our driver would stop at every single street corner and yell out, "Orascom!" at anybody who was standing nearby. That was the name of the place we were looking for, and at each corner some local would point down a block or two and maybe indicate a turn or two as well. When we would arrive there would be nothing and we'd go through the whole thing again. "Orascom!" After driving around forever we finally stumbled upon it.

Inside we found the office we needed and stood in the entry waiting for somebody to acknowledge us. We stood and stood until another customer came along and motioned us to follow him. There were three employees in the place but nobody said a word to any of us. After a few minutes a boy came in and took coffee orders from the five customers now sitting inside. After polishing off our coffee we still hadn't spoken to anybody.

Finally, after at least half an hour, a guy who seemed to be the boss arrived and got down to business. We asked him about our part and he told us that unfortunately he was not the Volvo supplier. Apparently the Volvo website and the Red Sea guidebook were both wrong on this account. He did however give us the phone number we needed.

When we asked if it would be possible for him to call for us, he simply said no. Fortunately one of the other customers was a friendly guy who spoke some English. He grabbed the phone number and made that call, plus half a dozen other phone calls around town for us trying to track down our prop. Somehow in the end we had our parts ordered from the supplier, and they were set to arrive in a week.

WE SPENT THE REST OF THE DAY just wandering around the city. Cairo obviously sees plenty of tourists, so we walked around in total anonymity, only occasionally being hit up by a tout for one thing or another.

We visited the Cairo Tower. It seems every city in the world has a tower, and we took the lift to the top of this one. Cairo spread out in every direction and went on forever. We could just barely make out the three pyramids of Giza through the thick pollution haze hanging over the city. It was still enough to get us excited about visiting.

Finding a beer in Cairo can be a bit of a challenge. You can of course get one in all the major hotels, but that isn't much fun. We eventually found a small café in which Saddam Hussein used to booze it up when he was in town. These days there are no dictators hanging around and instead just a handful of tourists straggle in out of the heat looking for a Stella.

Stella is an Egyptian beer brewed since 1897. Ali and I are trying to make sense of a country that can brew a beer for over a hundred years but still make us sit in a back room to drink it. For all the history in the place, it was certainly lacking in ambience; and after one quick Stella, we were back out on the streets.

MAY 10, 2006: PORT GHALIB, EGYPT

We made it back to *Bum* after an interesting overnight bus ride. Yesterday at four o'clock, after eleven days, we received our prop. We excitedly headed straight to the bus station to find out what time we would be heading home. Unfortunately the ticket girl told us the bus wasn't expected until eleven p.m.

Here in Egypt there is some sort of strange rule in effect that foreigners are only supposed to ride on specific buses traveling in a police-escorted convoy. That would have been the eleven o'clock bus. We asked her what time the local bus ran and she said six. There is a little known loophole that says foreigners can travel on the local buses as long as there are less than four of them onboard. Apparently this is all in an attempt to keep deaths of tourists to a minimum in case of a terrorist act. An entire busload of dead Westerners can have a bit of a negative impact on the almighty tourism dollar, while the death of just four will only make headlines for a day. Anyway, we got tickets for the local bus at six and crossed our fingers.

Everything was going smoothly enough. The bus left pretty close to its scheduled time, and the two large men in front of us had graciously brought their seats all the way forward, which allowed me to almost fit my legs in the seat.

Then three hours into our twelve-hour journey, the bus suddenly screeched to a halt on the shoulder. The bus driver's assistant jumped off, ran to the back, and opened up the engine compartment. The next thing we heard was, "Narrrrrr!" followed by a scream from the back of the bus and a stampede towards the door. We hustled off the bus with the rest of the crowd, eventually realizing that *narr* meant fire.

Outside the bus we learned that the fire was more of a flicker and it was quickly extinguished, though not before melting a few important engine bits. The men made a line along the shoulder to relieve themselves and then began chain smoking. Nobody seemed too concerned.

We thought at that point that there wasn't a single English speaker on the bus, but then a guy approached us and said in halting English that they were sending a replacement bus, hopefully arriving in three hours. A bus did eventually arrive to pick us up and after just a few hours delay we were on our way again.

Back at the marina we found *Bum* looking really sad. There had obviously been a dust storm or two and she was completely covered in dirt. The dinghy was totally flat but still floating somehow, like a big dirty garbage bag. Our Egyptian flag had torn loose and was flapping wildly by one corner. Overall she looked like she had been abandoned years earlier, not eleven days.

EGYPT HAD IT ALL. *We absolutely loved it. There is simply no other place like it on earth, with the pyramids, tombs, mummies, and the mosques. We did our best to take it all in. Meanwhile the people were simultaneously both the best and the worst part of Egypt, which I suppose could be said for just about any country.*

One day a local would pick us up as we hitchhiked down the road, deliver us to our door, and not accept a penny in compensation. The next day our cabbie would drive us the long way around the city trying to pawn us off on his huckster camel tour buddies. One minute a local man would give Ali his seat on a bus, and the next she'd be receiving lewd catcalls. Our experiences really ran the gamut. But through it all, we were overwhelmed by the kindness and the generosity of the people.

In the end it took eleven days for our prop to arrive, much longer than we had anticipated. However it all worked out for the best. We really felt as if we got to know Cairo and understand a little better how the place worked. By the time we left, we had grown accustomed to its crowded city streets, hectic markets, and even its stifling polices on alcohol.

After returning from Cairo we quickly decided we wanted to see more. There was still a lot to see in the southern part of the country. By now we had mastered the transportation system, so getting around wouldn't present any problems. In one afternoon between our boat and Luxor we hitchhiked, took a bus, a share taxi, and rode a train. We then spent another week visiting more amazing sites before forcing ourselves back to the boat to put the last of the Red Sea behind us.

MAY 22, 2006: PORT GHALIB, EGYPT

Today I was reading an issue of Latitudes & Attitudes magazine. It is no wonder that people think we are crazy for doing this. I honestly cannot stand to read these sailing magazines anymore. They are so full of horror stories and ridiculous tips from the pros that I can't help but roll my eyes and laugh.

Lats & Atts is supposed to be the fun, don't take yourselves too seriously cruising magazine. Yet they are just as bad as the rest of them. First off, they fill a page every month with a piracy report, which in the dozens of magazines I've seen has never contained one incidence of a cruising sailboat being attacked. The latest issue talks about a cargo ship in Bangladesh being followed by three boats filled with robbers that never came closer than fifty meters away. Ooooh, that's scary news for cruisers. Seriously, what does that have to do with cruising?

Then there is an article by a guy that I just really can't understand. In order, the article talks about how he absolutely would not let Jamaican authorities confiscate his 9mm handgun while he visited their country, how he scared off an alleged mugger by brandishing a collapsible baton which he just happened to have handy, and how finally, at the end of the day, he had a conversation with friends in which he said, "We couldn't understand how the world could be so crazy and full of violence. I still don't understand to this day."

Umm, don't you think maybe it has something to do with people carrying 9mm handguns and collapsible batons with them wherever they go? What's the old saying? Go looking for trouble and trouble will find you.

The next article was about spare parts. If we had packed even a third of these "essential" spares on our boat, we would have sunk right there at the dock in Florida. The first six in the list constitute an entire engine as a spare. Then of course you need five rebuild sets for each toilet onboard. Five! That would mean ten toilet rebuild kits for us. How about one rebuild kit, a bottle of Pepto Bismol, and a handful of Tums instead.

You also need three of every size and type of screwdriver. Very good advice since apparently screwdrivers can't be found anywhere outside of the United States. Hardware stores in Tonga only contain bamboo sticks and nails made of seashells. No, I swear. Bring as much black electrical tape as you can carry. Again, this must not be available anywhere else. Thankfully, I'm still on my first roll. Instant glue. Well, alright I'll give the author that one. As far as I'm concerned nobody can ever have too much super glue.

The list has a total of forty-five items to check off and then at the end states, "This is of course just a partial list." Well I must say, Ali and I are in a whole lot of trouble. Considering that we could only check off four items on this partial list of necessary spare parts and tools, I'm not so sure we should go any farther.

It's no wonder the average boat owner never leaves the dock. According to the magazines, we are all under-prepared for the horrific dangers in store for us out at sea. What horrific dangers? Well you have to read the books to learn what those are.

MAY 24, 2006: EL GOUNA, EGYPT

Yesterday, after waiting for what felt like forever, our weather window finally appeared and we were on our way north. It was just over a hundred miles to our next stop, a quick overnight sail. The forecast showed nothing over five knots, so we were a little disappointed when we found we had fifteen knots out of the north.

At around two a.m. the wind had died down to only five knots and we were looking forward to an early morning arrival. Then, while Ali slept, I watched the wind climb steadily from five, to fifteen, to twenty-five, to thirty. Before the waves even had a chance to build I turned the boat straight west towards shore and a Plan B anchorage.

Ali took over at four and then woke me awhile later to discuss our options. We were getting close to land and the waves had flattened out, however the wind was still howling. We decided to press on to our original destination, turning north again and sticking close to shore on an inside passage between the reefs.

It was only an overnight passage, but we were proud of ourselves for managing to sail nearly the entire way in pretty strong winds without actually beating on the boat or ourselves, thus maintaining our ability to say to other cruisers, "No, we've hardly had to beat at all. The Red Sea has been a piece of cake." Which is always fun since, after all, cruising is a competition.

MAY 28, 2006: SINAI PENINSULA COAST, EGYPT

Right now we are sitting at anchor in Mersa Hammam, just fifty miles south of the Suez Canal, having a tea, watching the sunrise, listening to the wind howl past at thirty knots, and watching dozens of flies bounce off the door while trying to get inside the boat with us. It's lovely.

We left yesterday morning bound for Suez. Our weather forecast looked absolutely perfect once again with not a hint of wind over ten knots. We hadn't seen a cloud in weeks and today was no different. The wind was close to what was predicted and we motorsailed through the reefs, around dozens of oil rig platforms, and across the shipping lanes to the west coast of the Sinai Peninsula.

We stuck close to shore so we'd have a place to hide in case of a sudden weather change. Things looked good as I woke Ali up for her first watch of the night with our speed at over six knots and the wind at only five. She woke me three hours later with our speed down to two knots and the wind up to twenty-five. I don't know why she does that.

As the sun came up we were able to turn back towards land and hug the coast. Once we got to shore things were quite a bit better with the waves beaten down by the shallow water and the winds slightly less because of the mountains lining the coast. By early afternoon we dropped the anchor out front of Mersa Hammam, a stark, abandoned place, with enough half-built housing onshore to shelter a thousand families.

Not long after settling in, we had some visitors come by on a fishing boat. They saw our outboard and seemed excited as they tried to explain to me the part they needed. Like everybody does when speaking to somebody who doesn't understand their language, these guys just repeated themselves over and over, louder and louder.

Seeing as our Arabic is limited pretty much to hello and no thank you, we didn't have much luck. I think I eventually got the point across that we didn't have any spare parts for the motor, just the motor itself. I was then able to explain much more easily that we didn't smoke cigarettes, and they were off.

At two this morning I made the mistake of waking up and having a look around outside. The wind was down to ten knots and things felt pretty good. I woke Ali up and we quickly raised the anchor and got underway.

The anchorage was behind a flat spit of land and it didn't seem possible that the wind could be blocked by anything, especially since it hadn't been the day before when we came in. But sure enough, ten minutes after motoring out the wind was at twenty knots, and ten minutes after that it was whipping our faces at thirty. We pressed on, pounding through the waves for over an hour before admitting defeat and turning around. It only took us thirty minutes to fly back to the anchorage downwind and by four o'clock we were back in bed sound asleep as if nothing had happened.

MAY 29, 2006: SINAI PENINSULA COAST, EGYPT

We woke up this morning to fifteen knots of wind and decided to just go for it. About three miles out, the wind had kicked up to thirty knots and it was feeling like an instant replay of the day before. The difference was that today it was light out so we could see just how bad the conditions were. Surprisingly, even with the strong winds, they weren't too bad at all. We spent the day tacking offshore, then back inshore, with a little motoring up the coast thrown in, and by early afternoon we were safely anchored just twenty-five miles short of the canal.

Lately we have hit one of those rough patches in our trip where nearly everything on the boat seems to fall apart at the same time. Every single passage, no matter how short, sees at least three more minor things breakdown.

In just the last month, we have had the prop fall off, had a problem with the starter battery, found a fourth crack in the dinghy davits, had a water leak through the port rudder post, and two hatches have started leaking again. Then in the last three days, the stern rubrail has fallen off, all the fuel filters had to be replaced as the dirty fuel was choking our engines, and the bows are covered in oil courtesy of the rigs chugging away along the coast. Then, of course, there is the ever-present dinghy leak. Seriously, if we ever get the urge to go sailing again after this trip, I hope we'll read this and charter a boat instead.

MAY 30, 2006: SUEZ CANAL, EGYPT

Yet another early start this morning. It was still dark out at five a.m. as we got the boat ready to go; start the computer, plug in the GPS, and warm up the engines. It was a beautiful morning, and we were soon underway.

The wind was steady at twenty knots and coming straight out of the north again. There is no doubt that we have tacked more in the last two days then we have in the last two years. By eleven we were at the canal, just in time to follow a northbound convoy of ships in on our way to the Suez Canal Yacht Club. Yacht club is a pretty fancy name for what this place really is, a boarded-up building with a bunch of moorings out front of it.

The agent we had hired to perform the Canal transit paperwork had apparently been calling on the VHF for us for two days and was happy when we finally answered him this morning. We told him our VHF had been on the fritz, but the truth is we just never have it turned on. Our agent and his helpers were on hand to help us tie the boat up between the moorings.

All secured, he came aboard and informed us that we would be going through the canal tomorrow. Apparently the British Navy is coming through within the next few days and yachts aren't allowed to transit at the same time as warships. In fact a few yachts were stuck here today because of the U.S. Navy submarine that came through this afternoon. That was pretty cool to see. The sub cruised by, practically submerged just a hundred yards away with a group of officers standing on top of it. There was a helicopter escorting it through, as well, which circled over and fired off a few rounds right in front of us just in case we had any bad intentions.

We still had about a hundred dollars worth of Egyptian pounds on us and figured that Israel might not be overly anxious to exchange them for us, so we decided to head to town and replenish our food stocks with it. It's a good thing too, as we were completely out of Twinkies and down to our last strawberry soda.

With the money spent, we headed back to the boat and worked on some fun projects there. Things like trying to remove oil sludge and seal up dinghy leaks. After that Ali warmed up some sausages and burnt some pancakes for dinner before we called it a night. We've got a big day of canal transiting ahead of us tomorrow.

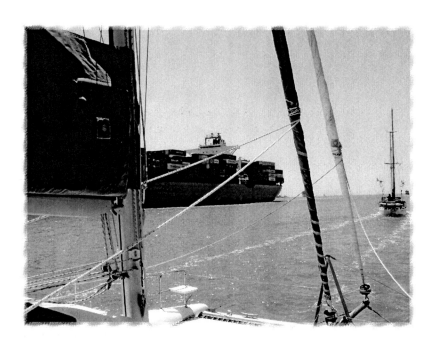

MAY 31, 2006: SUEZ CANAL, EGYPT

What more could a girl want than to have her husband take her, along with one Egyptian stranger, on a trip through the Suez Canal for their wedding anniversary? Ali's a lucky girl indeed.

By eleven o'clock all of our canal transit dues had been paid and we had our passports and clearance papers in hand. Shortly after, our pilot arrived and we were on our way. It was time to put another cruiser myth to the test. Cruiser folklore states that Suez Canal pilots are pigs and that you can expect your transit of the canal to be the least enjoyable experience of your sailing life. Poop smeared walls and cigarette burns on your gelcoat are apparently the norm. We had heard fourth hand or read these stories a hundred times.

Of course this turned out not to be the case. Our pilot was harmless, lounging around in the cockpit while I drove the boat and Ali played her role as the subservient housewife. It's a role she doesn't often play, much to my chagrin, but sometimes it's just easier to go along. The canal itself is really about the least interesting stretch of water imaginable. It is so uninteresting in fact that our pilot even fell asleep for an hour. Low sandy hills stretched forever while we tooled along through our little creek in the middle of it all.

Our pilot didn't really do a thing. Ali asked him not to smoke in the cockpit, which he didn't, he only accepted one can of pop and one aspirin, and he barely ate any of the snacks we put out for him. He hardly talked to us at all, but he sure did love to chat on the VHF, which is what he spent most of the day doing. That was just fine with us.

At one point a group of fishing boats was passing us and our pilot asked if we had some bottles of water for them. We told him no, figuring that saying yes would only lead to more handout requests, and he relayed the information to them. They didn't seem happy about that, but our pilot didn't press us about it either. He asked us to go a little faster as well, but we were running the engines as hard as we wanted to already, so again we just said no, and that was the end of that. Overall it was just a long boring day of motoring through uninspiring landscape with an uninteresting stranger lying in our cockpit.

Eight hours later we rolled into Ismalia, a small town at the halfway point of the canal where sailboats have to spend the night. Ismalia was also where we dropped off our pilot and played out the *baksheesh* game.

About an hour before we got in our pilot asked me if I would have a present for him and then proceeded to tell me all about his wife and three children. So when we finally got in and tied up I was ready for him. I handed him $10 U.S. dollars and a couple packs of smokes. From the look on his face you'd have thought that I had just set a dog turd in his hand.

No big surprise there, it's part of the game. We already knew that $10 was more than generous. In fact even our Egyptian agent had recommended $5-10 as a good tip. Our pilot asked us to double his *baksheesh*, we said no. He asked for five more, we said no. Out of options he turned and climbed off the boat without saying goodbye or thank you. It was a little disappointing since we had been so pleased with how the day went, but we quickly got over it.

JUNE 2, 2006: SUEZ CANAL, EGYPT

The next day we got a late start after having spent the morning making dozens of phone calls trying to track down our new pilot. He finally arrived and we got underway around noon. We knew we would be pushing our arrival by leaving that late but had no reason to hang around Ismalia.

Our pilot was a good guy. He was a Muslim who repeatedly performed his ablutions, cleansing his arms, hands, and face in our bathroom before coming out on deck to wash his feet with a glass of water and say his prayers. As far as piloting, he took his job a little too seriously, insisting on sitting next to me for hours on end. The only time he left me was for prayer. Praise Allah for those breaks.

The day passed utterly uneventfully. The Suez Canal is not an exciting place to motor through. There are no locks, and nothing to look at other than the next channel marker a quarter mile away, all day, for forty-five miles.

Because we left so late, the currents were against us nearly the entire time. We finally rolled into Port Said at eight o'clock, just as the sun was disappearing. That's when things got interesting.

PORT SAID IS AN ABSOLUTELY filthy shipping port. The waterfront is littered with rusting buoys and boats, while the channel is clogged with cargo ships, ferries, and pilot launches. We asked our pilot where we could anchor but he assured us there was no place to go other than the yacht club. The yacht club was just a small break in the middle of the general congestion where we could drop the anchor and tie up two stern lines to a decrepit wall. At this point, with dark setting in, we didn't have much choice.

A boat arrived to pick up our pilot just as we were trying to maneuver into position to drop our anchor. We handed our pilot a bag with a couple t-shirts, a cap, and ten bucks. He grabbed it and immediately started sifting through it. He must have been happy because he didn't ask for more. Nor did he bother to say thank you, something we had long ago given up hearing in Egypt. Then, like a little kid on Halloween he snuck off to the side of the boat, opposite the pilot boat that was picking him up. Hidden, he started stuffing his goods into his empty briefcase, which had been brought along specifically for that purpose.

Meanwhile Ali and I were scrambling around trying to keep our boat from bashing into giant steel moorings and the pilot boat. We finally yelled to our pilot to get off our boat and he responded by asking for *baksheesh* for the pilot boat guys. As if they had done us some giant favor. By this point we were yelling at the pilot boat to come get him off, which they finally did while simultaneously asking for *baksheesh* themselves. Our boats continued to bounce in the wake just inches away from each other. They finally left empty handed, allowing us to finish getting anchored and tied off to the wall.

Our plan was to spend the night there and leave by five a.m. The reason for that is that it is illegal to arrive in Israel at night, which is what would have happened if we left right then.

As soon as we were tied up, the guy who had helped us with our lines told us that we would need a pilot the next day to take us the rest of the way out of the harbor, approximately a half mile. Cost: twenty-six dollars. Fine, whatever, we just wanted to go to bed. Then he told us the marina fee was fifteen dollars for the night. That would make this crappy, filthy, cockroach infested cement wall the most expensive marina in all of Egypt. We told him no way, we would pay him eight, and we would want a receipt. He told us he would get his boss then.

In the meantime, I dropped our dinghy down because it had sprung a massive leak earlier in the day. It was obvious that a new seam had opened up because there wasn't a breath of air left inside of it. When it is that flat it is impossible to keep it tied up tightly and it swings wildly, which then makes the dinghy davits that hold it crack even worse than they already are.

Just as I set about fixing that, the boss came over. He asked how long we were, and I told him ten meters. He thought for a minute and then said, "The cost is $1.50 per meter, so $15."

Amazing, that was exactly the same cost the kid had come up with without even knowing the length of our boat. He said we must pay this and the $26 pilot fee to him right away or else we must leave.

We asked, "If we leave now we don't need a pilot?"

He said he wouldn't even report that we had stopped there. The group that had gathered around were all kind of snickering, thinking that they had us screwed over because it was so dark now that there was no way we would leave.

But we said, "Okay we're out of here then, thanks for all your help."

Now it is pitch black except for the lights of the city and there were still ships all over the place, but none of them seemed to be moving any longer. We had a quick look at the charts and thought we spotted a basin that we would be able to anchor in. However, when we got close we found that there was a huge ship in it and someone on deck yelling at us to get the hell away from them.

Back on the charts, we realized that if we went outside Port Said into the open ocean the water was still shallow enough to anchor. We followed the channel out and motored another half mile or so before turning outside the shipping channel into the shallow Mediterranean water. We made sure to get far enough away that we wouldn't be run over in the middle of the night.

Fortunately the wind had died and there was only a tiny swell rolling through. By ten o'clock our anchor was down and I went back to work on the dinghy, managing to quickly find the new leak and get it super glued in the dark. Ali whipped up our first meal of the day, peanut butter toast, and we fell into bed exhausted at midnight.

JUNE 3, 2006: HERZLIYA, ISRAEL

Considering where we were anchored, it was a miracle that we had such a great night of sleep. The wind stayed calm, and once the ships stopped moving around, the sea went flat. For about the tenth morning in a row we were up at the crack of dawn and on our way, sailing in the Mediterranean Sea at last. We had nice downwind sailing all day until at dark when the wind died away completely, leaving us to motor through the night towards Israel.

Israel has some strict security precautions in place, which for us meant that we were required to call them on the VHF upon arriving within fifty miles of their coast. We didn't make contact at fifty miles, or forty miles for that matter; but around thirty-five miles out, we started to hear back from them. Our connection was terrible, and we spent pretty much the entire morning trying to hear and understand each other. We know that our VHF doesn't work very well, it never has, but we use it so rarely that we have never bothered to try and fix it. Now for the first time, it was a real pain in the ass.

After a few hours, we thought things were pretty well squared away. Right up until a Navy patrol boat came roaring towards us from out of nowhere. They kept their big guns trained directly on us while we once again relayed all of our information. They told us to call yet another station to report the same information a third time. We never really did get through to that station, however, and eventually just gave up.

When the Navy boat was alongside of us they yelled over in their loudspeaker, "How are you?" Not having any other way to reply, we gave them the thumbs up. Then, not five minutes later, Ali was reading our guidebook which said, "Any gesture in which the thumb is extended is considered offensive, so avoid giving thumbs up." Not even on land yet, and we'd already committed a faux paux.

At noon we arrived in Tel-Aviv Marina. We were met by two guys from Israeli Security who poked around the boat a bit before handing over control to the lady in charge. She came aboard and sat us down for an interview. She poured through our passports, asking if we had any family in any of the Middle Eastern countries we had recently visited, or if anybody could have gotten aboard and planted a bomb while we were away from the boat.

After the interview it was her turn to poke around inside and swipe some bomb/drug detectors all over everything. She sent those away and then asked us to show her our Israel guidebook. That request surprised us, but she seemed satisfied when she saw that we had a bunch of stuff highlighted, thus proving that we planned to do a little touring and not just blow ourselves up on a crowded bus.

Our drug screen came back negative, and we were handed over to one last police lady who had us fill out our visas. She then asked if we wanted our passports stamped. We regretfully declined, since we weren't sure where our travels might end up taking us. A few Muslim countries refuse admittance to anybody with an Israeli stamp in their passport.

Anyway, I make light of the security screening but they've obviously got good reason for it. They were all very friendly during the whole thing and were really happy to welcome us to their country. And best of all, not a penny exchanged hands.

We had originally planned to stay in the Tel-Aviv Marina; but once we saw how ridiculously crowded it was, we decided to head five miles farther up the coast to Herzliya where there is a huge new marina. By law we have to stay in a marina while here in Israel.

After arriving in Herzliya, Ali and I went straight to work washing the boat of tons of African sand. It felt like a brand new home once that was done. We celebrated by walking the hundred meters to the McDonald's in the shopping mall that is overlooking the marina. This is where we got our first taste of Mediterranean Europe prices. Big Mac combo, nearly eight bucks. A few celebratory drinks after dinner and we ended a very long couple of days.

WE HAD MIXED FEELINGS *about being in the Med. It seemed to surprise a lot of people that the leg between Oman and Egypt was our favorite part of our trip to that point. It was so much more interesting than anywhere else we'd been.*

Throughout that area of the world, we got the chance to meet people who were so unlike us. Yet, at the same time, we were all very much the same. People everywhere just want to be happy and to surround themselves with family and friends. These people invited us into their homes, made sure our buses got us where we needed to go, and helped us find the things we needed to continue on.

"Ahhhmereeeka! Welcome to our country!" We must have heard that a thousand times after being asked where we were from. Where was all the angry shaking of fists and stone throwing? It didn't take long to understand that people have no problem differentiating the politics of a country from the people of a country.

It was so much fun to travel in a place where we stood out as being different. In the South Pacific we were generally treated as just another tourist to the locals. In New Zealand and Australia we appeared no different until we opened our mouths to speak. In SE Asia there seemed to be little interest in us. But from the moment we stepped foot in the Middle East, we were a novelty.

Most people were so amazed that we were in their country that all they wanted to do was make sure we had the best experience we could, so that we'd walk away with a good impression of their home. We went into that area of the world not sure what to expect. The media certainly didn't give us a good impression, but we came out of each country blown away by the incredible people we met along the way. The Red Sea region has definitely become a highlight of our journey.

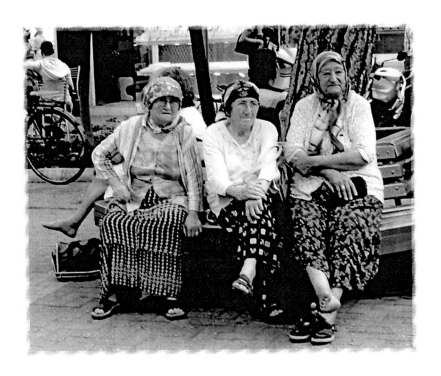

JUNE 9, 2006: HERZLIYA, ISRAEL

A convoy of cruisers has arrived over the last couple days. Cruisers with an insatiable appetite for information. Almost before they were done docking, they began asking questions. What are the showers like? Is there a laundry? How do you get downtown? Is the food safe to eat? Where is a good restaurant?

My favorite was when they started questioning us about an ATM. Remember we are in Israel, in a marina that has a shopping mall towering over it. I think most people would conclude that there would be an ATM somewhere in the mall.

"How do you get money here?"

"Uhhh, ATM."

"Oh, really, where is that?"

"In that big shopping mall right there in front of you."

"Oh, I see. Where inside the mall?"

And on and on and on. Before this trip I thought cruisers were much more independent people, but the truth we've found is that they really like to stick together in groups, and that they need to have as much information as possible before attempting anything at all on their own. I'm trying not to pass judgment. I'm just saying that it has really surprised me. I realize it is the twenty-first century and we aren't exactly blazing new trails, but can't they at least pretend to be modern-day adventurers?

I HATE TO ADMIT IT, but upon our arrival in Israel, Ali and I were really ignorant of the country's politics. Our knowledge and understanding was probably increased ten-fold simply by reading our guidebook. Over the course of the next couple weeks we learned more than we ever would have by watching the nightly news.

As we do in just about every country, we rented a car. Being Americans we found it easy to drive all over the place, passing through checkpoints with hardly a sideways glance. Though Israeli tourism is heavily geared towards religion, Ali and I really enjoyed ourselves, visiting some incredibly sacred religious sites, while also floating on our backs and taking funny pictures in the Dead Sea. We stayed with a family that we had met back in the Galapagos Islands, even sleeping in their bomb shelter. Then one day we changed a flat tire right along the Syrian border just five feet from a sign warning us that off the road was a minefield. All reminders that this is a country that is constantly on edge.

After seeing much of the country on our own wheels, we hopped on a bus to take us to the border of Jordan. At the border our bus was held up for an hour while bus after bus filed past us. It wasn't until a friendly passenger explained to us that we were on a Palestinian-only bus that we understood what the hold up was all about.

In our brief visit to Israel, we didn't figure it all out but we did learn a lot about the amazingly diverse people who share the tiny country and call it home.

JUNE 18, 2006: HERZLIYA, ISRAEL

We're getting ready to leave again. We spent the morning at the grocery store where surprisingly we didn't buy one package of cookies. We did however load up on Skippy and are now looking forward to a passage filled with peanut butter toast. Being on our boat is like being in college again.

Drop off the rental car, wash the boat, fill the water tanks, hang up the dinghy, pay the marina bill, eat one last pizza with no meat, see a movie, and we are officially ready to cast off.

JUNE 20, 2006: EN ROUTE TO TURKEY

Underway again. We used to daydream about having a furling mainsail and imagine what great sailors we would be if we had one. No more of us being too lazy to raise the main. No sir, we'd be flying along harnessing the power of the wind. But after the last few thousand miles, we realize that what this boat really needs is bigger engines. Man, if only we had forty horses on each side instead of twenty. Yep, we'd be happy then, no more bitching and complaining coming from our mouths.

The point is that we never actually seem to sail our sailboat. We spent the afternoon moaning about our slow progress, motorsailing at three knots with just enough wind on the nose to chop up the water, but not enough to actually sail. Fortunately after nightfall the wind died away and left us to motor in peace.

The upside is that we are in the Mediterranean, and when we look at the chart it seems as if in just one sluggish day we've crossed half an ocean. Normally after a day like this we would look at the chart, of the Indian Ocean for instance, and it would seem like we hadn't moved at all. Now we look at the computer screen and we're practically in Turkey.

JUNE 22, 2006: EN ROUTE TO TURKEY

As has become our custom, we have now been motoring for forty-eight hours straight. We get a little bit of a head wind in the afternoon that we are able to motorsail with, but other than that it is just light winds and slow motoring. We haven't seen a dolphin, a flying fish, or even a bird since we left Israel, and we are starting to wonder if we are the last living things on earth. We'll find out in another day or two.

We ran out of propane today. We knew we were low but have been procrastinating on that project. So this morning Ali informed me I'd be getting nothing but peanut butter and jelly sandwiches for the next couple of days. That's alright, since I love PB&J, but Ali may kill me for not getting any coffee during that time.

JUNE 23, 2006: KAS, TURKEY

That was quite possibly the least eventful passage ever. Four days and three nights of steady motoring. But who cares? We're here and the boat is in one piece.

Kas is our first truly Mediterranean stop and it is exactly what we had envisioned. The little harbor is absolutely packed full of boats. We pulled in and motored carefully along the quay until we found a perfect opening. We dropped anchor and Med moored, backing our way in.

Within one minute of getting our lines tied off, another boat pulled in and began backing in next to us. The space looked big enough for a twelve foot dinghy, but this fifty-two footer just backed in and started pushing boats out of the way until we were all packed in nice and tight. Definitely something that is going to take some getting used to, but it works.

We got asked another strange cruiser question today. This is one that we've heard a lot in the last couple of years, ranking it second behind only, "So how long have you been out?"

Our neighbor on the fifty-two footer, immediately after getting settled in, turns to us and instead of saying, "Hey thanks," says, "So, is that *your* boat?" Making sure to heavily stress the "your" part of the question. I guess it's possible we could be crew, though I have yet to see a boat as small as ours with paid help onboard. This cruising world sure does have an elitist mentality.

The town of Kas begins right at the yacht quay where there are dozens of restaurants, a pedestrian mall area, and some souvenir shops. The town feels so stereotypically European. Narrow streets lined with little shops and two-story flats with old ladies hanging laundry on the balconies while the men sit at the restaurants downstairs drinking tea and playing backgammon.

JUNE 25, 2006: KAS, TURKEY

Kas is a great place, the perfect start to our Turkish cruising. Yesterday we had a full day that started out early with a walk around town looking for coffee. There are probably close to a hundred restaurants in town and yet at nine a.m. not one of them was open. Mediterranean time is much different than we are used to.

Ali displayed her OCD soon after by putting us to work washing the boat. If there is a freshwater tap within reach, then we must wash. Already clean or not, it makes no difference. After that it was time to cool off, so we walked down the street to the beach. There aren't any actual beaches, but they have built terraces in the rocks around one area of the harbor and roped it off for swimming. The terraces are owned by different restaurants and each have laid out hundreds of chairs and umbrellas all over the cliffs, yet amazingly they don't bother us to buy anything. If we do, great; if not, enjoy the swim.

Anyway, we've really enjoyed our first taste of Turkey. The people have been terrific, going out of their way to help us out, and even store employees and restaurant waiters seem to take pride in doing a good job, which is something we're not necessarily used to seeing.

Then early this morning, a man was tooling along on his scooter throwing bags of fresh bread into each of the yachts along the quay. Ali was awake and he just handed her a bag with a smile and a nod. Of course there was a restaurant business card in the bag, but why be cynical?

UNFORTUNATELY THE REST OF THE COUNTRY didn't live up to our day one experience. Turkey was reported to be a cruiser's playground, which in retrospect should have set off all sorts of alarms in our heads. By this point we knew that when a place was popular with the cruising masses, we would almost undoubtedly not like it.

There wasn't just one thing that turned us off though. It was more a combination of factors. First and foremost was just how crowded the coast was. Every bay we visited was packed to the gills with yachts. The majority were large wooden day-charter yachts, filled with Europeans on holiday. There were hundreds, if not thousands, cruising the coast.

Then there were the towns. From Kas westward the place became more and more touristy and less and less Turkish. By the time we reached Marmaris we'd seen enough sunburned Brits to last a lifetime.

A couple of road trips redeemed the country somewhat though. There are all sorts of incredible ruins and archaeological sites around Turkey, most of which we found to be completely empty. We stood in a Roman amphitheatre perched on a cliff at the top of a mountain and couldn't see any sign of life in any direction. It was one of the most dramatic sites we'd ever visited and we had it all to ourselves.

The final straw was drawn the day our boat was broken into and robbed while we sat on a friend's boat a hundred yards away. We wanted nothing more at that point than to simply move on. But before we could leave we needed to do some boat work. We desperately needed a fresh bottom painting.

That's when we found out why cruisers love Turkey. It's not because the cruising is so good, it's because not cruising is so cheap. The coast is lined with government-owned marinas charging as little as five dollars a day. Hell, even if your entire retirement income came from social security you'd still be able to live happily here. And one visit to the marina pool in the afternoon showed that many a foreign cruiser was doing just that. After seeing that, we didn't feel guilty any more for not enjoying our cruise of the coast. No cruisers were. They were enjoying the "cruising" life in what was essentially a five dollar a day retirement community.

AUGUST 1, 2006: BODRUM, TURKEY

In the morning we are clearing out of Turkey. I hate to say it, but we're happy to do so. We just didn't find anything about cruising the Turkish coast appealing. It was like driving down the freeway and then trying to find a parking space at the shopping mall. The scenery was okay, and the water was clear, but the bays were so unbelievably crowded and the towns so touristy that we felt more like we were in Disneyland than Turkey. We did enjoy our road trip and our visit to Istanbul which makes me think that if we were ever to return to Turkey we'll stay as far away from the coast as possible.

Oh well, we can't expect to love every place we visit on a trip like this. Just look at the Marquesas. One thing is for sure, I would have never thought we'd be in Turkey saying we wished that we were back in Yemen instead.

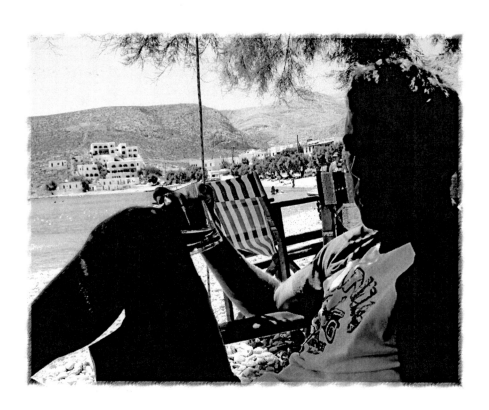

personal space

After the shortest distance we've ever traveled between two countries, eight miles, we found ourselves in Greece yesterday afternoon. Clearing out of Turkey was easy enough once everybody finally showed up for work. Clearing into Greece was a different story.

After tracking down the first office just fine and receiving their paperwork, I set out to find the customs officer. This took nearly two hours as I was sent from one end of town to the other a half dozen times. I eventually found him though, and he seemed like a nice guy who was going to bang out my paperwork and send me on my way. But then he asked for my boat registration, the one truly official piece of paper showing the boat is ours.

This is the routine in every country in the world, but here we suddenly had a problem. He looked at the copy I handed him, crumpled it up in his hand and spat on it. Or at least he made that fake spitting motion that people do in the movies to show their disgust with something. He apparently was not happy with just a copy and wanted the original.

I explained that we'd been sailing for three years and the original was at home in the United States. He didn't like this at all and asked how I was going to prove that the boat was mine. I told him he could look at my passport which was full of *Bumfuzzle* references and I also had other papers here that I could show him. "All copies!" he yelled out.

At this point I was still half expecting him to break out laughing and say he was just joking, but he was totally serious. He told me to go back to the boat and return with some official papers proving my ownership.

I went back to the boat and told Ali the story. She dug through our paperwork and pulled out the bill of sale and a couple of other closing documents. I spat on them and yelled, "All copies!" She thought that was funny, but still couldn't track down any originals. With my new copies I headed back in.

I tracked customs down once again, this time at a different office. Now there were three of them; the good cop, the bad cop, and the grinning sidekick. I produced the latest copies for their inspection. The original officer looked totally unimpressed with these papers as well, but fortunately a new guy took over the proceedings and acted a bit more lenient.

He flipped through all the papers, nodding thoughtfully, and then made a call to their superior to explain the situation. Obviously the superior couldn't have cared less, because the phone call lasted just fifteen seconds before my paperwork was being processed. Minutes later I shuffled out of the office with only one stop to go.

When I arrived at the port police to meet my final official, the first thing he asked me for was my boat registration. I handed him the copy and he asked, "Where is the original?" I turned around fully expecting to find two people standing there, one with a camera, and one white haired man with a microphone. This had to be *Candid Camera*.

But there was nobody behind me, and this guy was as serious as the last. I explained that I had just spent the past couple hours with customs going over this very issue and showed him my other copies. Somehow I persuaded him to believe it was my boat. He stamped my papers and we were officially cleared into Greece.

There was nothing left to do after that but to collect Ali and deposit ourselves at one of the harbor front *tavernas* for a few Mythos beers. Kos is only a few miles from Turkey, and it is really geared towards tourists as well, but it's got a much better vibe. Much more chill, for lack of a better word.

AUGUST 5, 2006: KOS, GREECE

After a couple of days on the, shall we say, very European beaches of Kos, we're moving on again. Here in Greece we have to check in and out of every single island that we visit. I figured after we were cleared into the country and had the transit log they required us to use, it would be an easy process, but I was wrong. They immediately asked for our original boat registration again and told us we could not leave the island until we had it.

So this morning, with the original paper in hand, we proceeded to the port police office again. We handed over the original registration, and a copy of our insurance. Greece is the first country we've visited that insists that we be insured. We, like at least half the cruisers out here, consider ourselves to be self-insured. However, a promise that we'll pay for any damage that we cause doesn't seem to cut it here.

Fortunately we foresaw that this was going to be a problem and we created our very own self-insurance company. We pay a deductible of $0 per month to ourselves in exchange for coverage equal to the amount of our bank balance. We even issued ourselves some insurance paperwork that looks pretty official and passed some very close scrutinizing by the Greek authorities. It's a good thing too, because one phone call to the number listed on our paperwork would have been answered by Ali's very confused sister, and would have probably landed us in Greek prison for ten to twenty.

Still, with our originals in hand, and our insurance papers cleared, the officer asked me for my captain's certificate. Keep in mind we have already been cleared into the country and are now just trying to sail from one island to another fifty miles away.

"Captain's certificate?" I asked.

"Yes."

"I don't have a captain's certificate."

"Oh boy. We've got a big problem then. How could you sail here without a certificate?"

"Nobody else has ever required one." I told her.

"But you are the captain, yes?"

"Yes."

"Then you must have a certificate. Stay here while I get my boss."

Luckily, as usual, the top officer didn't care about any of it and told her to finish my paperwork. Eventually we were cleared to proceed to the next island where presumably we will go through all of this again.

AUGUST 6, 2006: ASTYPALEA, GREECE

Early this afternoon we came around the corner of Astypalea Island and made our way through the miniscule entrance to Vathy Inlet. This bay is a mile long and a quarter mile wide, completely surrounded by scrubby hills, feeling just like an inland lake.

After the crowded anchorages of Turkey we couldn't believe this bay was empty. We picked a spot, which wasn't hard as it was just us, and dropped anchor.

We hadn't even finished setting the anchor when another sailboat came in behind us. They pointed their bow our way and came straight for us. Ali and I just stood there with our jaws wide open as they circled right next to us, dropped their anchor, and fell back directly alongside of us not fifty feet away.

Lately I feel like I'm always waiting for people to say, Just kidding! But they never do. So ten minutes after dropping our anchor in a mile long empty lake with a uniform twenty-five foot bottom we raised it, drifted back a ways and dropped the anchor again, reestablishing just a little bit of personal space.

AUGUST 8, 2006: ASTYPALEA, GREECE

After a night in our idyllic lake anchorage, we sailed to the other side of the island to check out the town of Astypalea. We could tell right away that we were going to like this place. It's a medium-sized town which climbs from the water straight up a hill that surrounds the castle standing at the top. It is the quintessential Greek island scene.

After anchoring we went in to have a look around and instantly fell in love. This really is everyone's vision of Greece. The hills are covered with white cube houses, blue shutters and doors and whitewashed stairways leading up to the top covered over with grapevines. Old men wearing fisherman's caps sit mending nets along the waterfront, and at the small beach in town dozens of kids play in the water. All of this is centered on a small bay with our boat anchored in the middle of it. It's truly perfect.

We picked a small restaurant with a view of everything, and over a lunch of spicy meatballs and cold beers watched the town go about its business. Later that night, back on the boat, the view was every bit as beautiful. The town's white buildings glowed against the dark hills while the well-lit castle stood watch over everything.

AUGUST 11, 2006: SANTORINI, GREECE

Earlier this afternoon we found ourselves cruising through a submerged caldera of a volcano, home to the biggest volcanic eruption in recorded history. So what in 1600 BC was a big round island is now moon shaped, with cliffs that rise straight up out of the water and tower hundreds of feet in the air.

Looking at our charts, I couldn't find any suitable anchorages as the cliffs hit the water and continue straight down a few hundred feet further. It looked like there might be a tiny shallow area near the town of Oia so we headed that way.

When we arrived at Oia we found that the town was actually located high above us at the top of the cliffs. As we got nearer we saw that there were two sailboats on moorings just off the shore and one of them was leaving. Realizing that there seemed to be no hope of anchoring anywhere inside the caldera we were relieved to be able to pick up the now vacant mooring.

The setting was spectacular. We need to crane our necks and look straight up in order to see the homes clinging to the cliffs high above us. Down at the waters edge there are just a couple of buildings, one of which is a small *taverna* that we quickly made our way over to.

The owner was a friendly fellow who was also the harbor master. He seemed completely unconcerned that we had picked up the mooring, indicating only that we pay him before we leave. His wife made us a nice home-cooked meal of pork *souvlaki* while we sat back and watched the occasional ferry boat pass by. The *taverna* was one of the greatest places we've been to relax, eat, drink Ouzo, and watch the world go by. At times like this, staring out at *Bum* on the water, we realize just how incredible this trip truly is.

AUGUST 12, 2006: SANTORINI, GREECE

For some reason we were surprised by how much we liked Oia. We climbed up the hill in the morning not really expecting much but somehow we spent the entire day walking around exploring the narrow passageways of another picture-perfect Greek town.

Back at the boat later on, we were talking about how much we were enjoying Greece, with its peaceful anchorages, good food, great towns, friendly locals, and relaxing atmosphere. The place almost seems too good to be true.

AUGUST 14, 2006: MILOS, GREECE

We had an easy motor over to Milos Island today. The town of Adamas is very quaint. We had a quick walk around, but it was scorching hot, it was Sunday, and about the only thing happening was the waterfront cafés. So once again we pulled up a couple of chairs to eat, drink, and watch the world go by. As we were sitting there I was thinking to myself, it seems like that is all we do here in Greece. Just then Ali said, "You know it seems like all we do here in Greece is eat, drink, and watch the world go by." We're clearly on the same wavelength.

But it's true, that is about all there is to do here. That, and go for a swim to cool off after doing all that sitting. Not that there is anything wrong with it, it's a great way to pass a day, a week, or more. And we're happy to do just that. In fact, looking around it seems that's all anybody is doing. We sat for hours and so did every other table around us.

AUGUST 16, 2006: KYTHIRA, GREECE

We just arrived in Kythira after a quick downwind, overnight passage. Yesterday we finished the clearing out of the country formalities, including going to the port police office to tell them we were leaving. The officer said, "Okay, no problem," and proceeded to wave us away. But we didn't think our next country would like seeing an entrance stamp for Greece with no exit stamp in our passports. We forced our way into the office and explained that we needed some sort of stamp and paperwork. He obligingly gave us what we wanted and told us to have a nice trip. Typical, that after the hassle in Kos with getting cleared in, that no other officer in the country cared one bit that we were there.

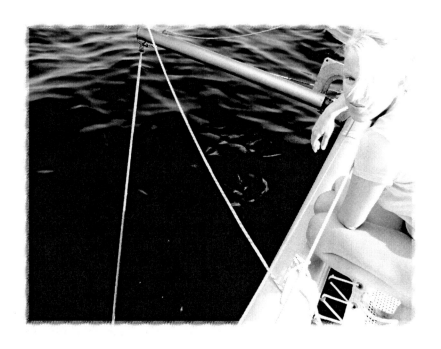

AUGUST 19, 2006: EN ROUTE TO MALTA

There is absolutely nothing happening out here in the Med. The wind has been more or less five knots for three days now, and we've been motoring steadily along the entire time. We read a book that talked about making this same passage and how they got plastered by the *meltemi*, a strong northwest wind that is supposed to be pretty much a daily occurrence in this part of the Mediterranean. Yet we haven't seen winds over ten knots in weeks.

AUGUST 21, 2006: VALETTA, MALTA

After another successful and simple passage in which we only turned off the engines for two hours, we arrived in Valetta, Malta. We found a spot at a marina right in the heart of the city, which is absolutely beautiful. The buildings, all of which look to be hundreds of years old, completely surround and tower over us.

Before doing anything, we gave the boat a good wash and are now off to have a walk around town to find customs and get checked in. We haven't had a chance to research Malta, so at this point we really have no plans, but from the looks of it there should be plenty to see.

MY MOM SURPRISED US *by flying out to meet us in Malta on just one day's notice. Together we explored the Maltese Islands, eating well, shopping, hanging out on the beach, and checking out dozens of museums and churches.*

Ali and I had originally planned to spend some time in Malta and then sail the short distance north to Italy. However after having a closer look at the map we decided that visiting Italy for a short period of time by boat wasn't going to allow us to see very much. In the end we left the boat in the Malta marina while we did a whirlwind tour of Italy.

It was a fun three weeks. We packed two backpacks and hopped the ferry to Sicily. From there it was trains and hostels through some of the world's most famous cities, which collectively hold both the world's most impressive historical artifacts, and its second greatest pizza. The pizza rivaled Chicago's, where it was invented around fifty years ago, an absolute fact that we learned while living there. The Italians seem to dispute this for some reason.

Leaning towers, Roman colloseums, Picassos, statues of David, canals, it all kept us happy and busy. It was a fun break; but by the time we returned to the boat, we couldn't wait to sleep in our own bed and were even looking forward to getting back out on the water. Life on land was wearing us out.

BY THIS POINT WE WERE OBSESSED *with travel. The sailing still hadn't really grown on us, but we loved the fact that we were sailing around the world. Breaks like this kept us excited and* motivated. Now, refreshed, we were ready to cross the Mediterranean. We knew it wouldn't be an easy trade wind passage, but after sailing this far we no longer had any concerns whatsoever. This was just what we did now. We crossed oceans.

SEPTEMBER 21, 2006: EN ROUTE TO SPAIN
We had meant to be on our way a couple of days ago but the weather was terrible. The wind was howling, and the waves crashing against the breakwall were huge. So instead we spent a couple of easy days around the boat and hanging out in Valetta.

We scored some duty-free fuel at a pittance compared to elsewhere in Europe. We also changed the oil and gave the boat one last good washing inside and out. This morning the weather finally turned, and we got underway again in calm conditions with only a bit of swell left over from the last week of strong winds.

SEPTEMBER 23, 2006: EN ROUTE TO SPAIN
After a couple of days with no wind, we have finally shut the engines off on day three with a nice eight knot breeze directly behind us. The passage has been pretty easy going so far. There has been a lot of shipping traffic but we haven't had to do much maneuvering.

The watermaker has been acting up today. It will be running just fine and then suddenly an error occurs. It seems the problem is air in the line, but I don't know why this would suddenly be happening. We bleed it at startup and then it runs for anywhere from five minutes to an hour before an error occurs again.

The dinghy is making trouble for us as well. The first day out it was leaking pretty bad, so we stopped the boat mid ocean, dropped it in the water and patched up two seams. The next day it was leaking again, a new spot that I was able to reach and patch while it was hanging up.

We've also had air in the fuel line on the port engine again. Not sure why this seems to happen so regularly on that engine, but I'm a professional fuel line bleeder now so it doesn't present much of a problem.

Other than that the boat seems to be running pretty well. A little overloaded with fuel and water at the moment which seems to be slowing us down a bit, but a couple more motoring days will take care of that.

SEPTEMBER 25, 2006: EN ROUTE TO SPAIN
The other day the wind showed up, and before we knew it we had thirty knots howling up behind us. Fortunately it was a straight downwind ride and wasn't too bad. Ali is no fan of the big following seas that look like they are going to swallow the boat whole, so she didn't care for these conditions much. But we did make good mileage with the sails triple reefed and flying wing-and-wing.

The boat handles those conditions amazingly well. I've read a lot of stories about people in monohulls who have to hand steer their boat whenever they are running directly downwind. Yet we never have to touch a thing, Bum just carves a nice straight line down the face of the waves, one after another with the autopilot humming away.

By dark on day four the wind had started to shift around, eventually putting itself on our nose. We tacked off and sliced through the waves, while the big seas flattened out and played catch up with the wind. By midnight the waves did just that, and we were pounding into twenty-five knots and big rolling seas. We both caught cat naps on the couch while the other one stood outside keeping an eye on everything.

Darkness also brought storms. We had lightning storms in every direction. Sometimes they were so intense they even lit up the pitch black sea, giving a quick glimpse of blue.

At one point I woke up to find Ali chanting, "I hate this, I hate it, I hate it, I hate it." That didn't seem like a very good mantra, so we tacked off and tried to calm things down a little bit.

By eight this morning conditions hadn't changed at all, and in fact were probably a little worse. I was sitting at the helm wearing the foul weather gear for only about the third time of our entire trip, getting absolutely soaked, when the idea to heave-to suddenly dawned on me.

We quickly cut the wheel hard over, backed the jib, let the main way out, and cranked the wheel all the way back over to the other side again. And just like that, it was total calm onboard. Twenty-five knots of wind whistling by, and big breaking waves rolling under us, but we were just bobbing up and down in peace. We could sit here for a week like this. That is, if we had any food, and our watermaker was working.

So here I sit typing away as if we were anchored in some extremely secluded bay. We have to remind ourselves to go outside every once in awhile to make sure no cargo ships are bearing down on us; but other than that, we just sit and wait for the wind and seas to calm down.

SEPTEMBER 27, 2006: EN ROUTE TO SPAIN

I don't know what our problem is, but this passage is turning out to be one of our hardest. It may be that we're just getting tired of passage making, because the conditions haven't really been all that trying. Or maybe it's the never-ending list of things that seem to go wrong on the boat that we just can't seem to solve. Whatever it is we are definitely looking forward to making landfall in a couple of days.

After eight hours of heaving-to the other day, the wind shifted rather dramatically in the right direction and even settled down under twenty knots. We got going and sailed for about an hour before the ugly weather surrounded us again. Dark clouds and rain were everywhere with just a doorway of blue sky in the middle. We pointed the boat for the blue and somehow made it through without getting rained on.

The wind had kicked back up over thirty knots, but we were moving the right direction. By evening though, the bashing had taken its toll on us and we were exhausted. We heaved-to once again while Ali made dinner and I tried to get some sleep. After a few hours the wind dropped and allowed us to get moving.

Not long after this our port engine really started to cause us headaches. There was air in the fuel line almost constantly, causing the engine to sputter and die. I'd bleed it and all would be fine for an hour, before it bogged out on us again. I've probably bled it ten times, and just as I was typing this, about to finally claim victory, I heard it start to hesitate again. It worked through the problem on its own this time, but I would guess that within an hour I'll be firing up the other engine and bleeding this one again. On the plus side, the watermaker is working. Apparently we've gotten the air out of that line. One out of two isn't bad I guess.

AFTER A DAY WITH TEN KNOT HEADWINDS yesterday, the wind finally gave up completely and we had calm today. It was a good thing since I spent the majority of it with my head in the port engine compartment. Ali even took the opportunity to whip up a batch of pudding. Guilt pudding.

Back in Malta we had bought a twelve-pack of little individual pudding containers. Yesterday I asked her where she put them and all I got in response was a sheepish look. Like a kid with her hand in the cookie jar. I had to laugh though because our food situation right now is truly pathetic. We are so uninterested in cooking that we left on this 1200 mile passage with essentially nothing to eat.

At the store, we bought two loaves of bread, pudding, and nacho chips. That's it, not even a fruit or vegetable. So who can blame a girl for eating the only sweet thing on the boat? Sadly, our saving grace has been the canned meatballs we stocked up on in Greece. We've made a meal out of those five nights out of seven so far.

This afternoon when I was filling up the fuel tanks, I did some calculating and realized that we were going to be about a hundred miles short of our destination unless we did some sailing soon. Unfortunately that isn't going to happen with no wind in the forecast for a couple more days at least. So now we've altered course to stop for fuel before carrying on to Malaga on the southern coast of Spain.

SEPTEMBER 30, 2006: COSTA DE SOL, SPAIN

That second day of calm weather we were supposed to have didn't happen. Instead we again found ourselves pounding head on into short seas. The wind was only twenty knots, but we were having a heck of a time pointing the boat anywhere near where we wanted to go.

On top of that we were having problems with the engine dying on us, and our charging system was malfunctioning. We were unable to charge the batteries for more than a few minutes before the battery alarm would start blaring and shut down the alternator. But just for a couple seconds at a time, beeeep, two seconds, beeeep, five seconds, beeeep.

With all of this happening, our mental health was quickly going downhill. Until finally, a breakthrough. While reading the troubleshooting section of my diesel maintenance book, I noticed a throwaway sentence right at the end. It said that if nothing else worked to check that the fuel tank vent hose wasn't blocked up. Problem solved.

While I was crawling around in the engine compartment I was staring at the alternator wiring wondering what could possibly be the problem. I noticed that the field wire from the alternator to the regulator had an extra four inch piece of wire spliced onto it, so instead of just one connection there were two, one of which had no real use. I grabbed my tools, cut off the extra piece, and reconnected the two ends. When we started the engine there was no more beeping. Cautiously, I claimed a second victory.

Yesterday morning we finally reached Spain. We were out of diesel with over two hundred miles to Benalmadena, where we are meeting family in just a few days. So even though what we really wanted to do was get off the boat, all we did was go into the marina, get diesel, a couple bags of chips for sustenance, and leave again.

About this time the engine started to sputter. I was devastated. I really thought I had it that time. I bled the fuel line yet again, but within an hour it was sputtering. Ali suggested I check the fuel vent hose again. I balked at the idea at first. We had been pounding into rough seas, but what were the chances that water had clogged up the hose again already?

Back into the engine compartment I went. I dutifully unhooked the hose and blew, not really believing that could be it. But Ali was right, water poured out the other end. A quick bleed and the engine was perfect again. Now I just have to figure out a solution to keep water out of that hose in the first place.

At the moment, we are still a hundred and fifty miles from the finish line, motoring at a pathetic three knots against a strong Strait of Gibraltar current, and directly into a little ten-knot wind kicking up just enough waves to keep the boat bouncing up and down uncomfortably. We're seriously going crazy. Maybe we should have spent a couple nights back at the marina.

TODAY THE WIND JUST WOULD NOT DIE down. It was forecast to be five knots but instead we had twenty-five on the nose. It feels as if it has been on our nose for a week straight. Our track hasn't exactly been the shortest route to our destination.

So when we finally reached the southeast tip of Spain and were about to go around it, into the Strait of Gibraltar, we decided instead to pull into the small bay and anchor for the night. We didn't have a chart for the area but it turned out to be perfect, well protected, shallow, and sandy. It felt great to drop the anchor and stop moving.

The problems weren't over yet though. While Ali was making dinner, the breaker for the propane popped. We reset it and it popped again. I went and emptied the chain locker, crawled inside and started poking around. I took a bottle of soapy water and sprayed all the fittings, immediately identifying the problem.

Our very rusty solenoid was leaking. I pulled the entire fitting apart, took the solenoid out of the middle, and reconnected the fitting without the solenoid. After another jury rigged bypass of a safety device, dinner was saved, along with our sanity. Sort of. We may have been better off without having another meal of meatballs and rice.

With a hundred miles to go, we are really hoping that tomorrow's weather forecast proves correct and we can finally finish this passage. We need to get there before something else on the boat breaks.

OCTOBER 1, 2006: COSTA DE SOL, SPAIN

Thankfully the weather cooperated and did what was predicted, which was to be very light and on the nose. We are now running a mile offshore along the southern coast of Spain. The view is beautiful, with layer after layer of mountain fading into the distance.

Unfortunately it looks like we're going to have to find ourselves a Volvo mechanic as soon as we can. I still haven't completely solved the port engine problem, and now the starboard engine is acting up. It's making a different sound, sort of a higher pitch than normal. It doesn't sound good and we are completely avoiding using that engine at this point. This passage included a long stretch of poor weather and the boat has taken some lumps because of it.

OCTOBER 4, 2006: DUQUESA, SPAIN

Things just do not want to improve for us. We finally beat our way into Benalmadena marina the other morning. The marina had not answered any of our e-mails but our cruising guide said they had one thousand berths, making them the largest marina we had ever visited. We weren't too concerned about them having space available.

Turns out we should have been. They looked at me like I must be crazy when I strolled into the office and told them we'd like to stay a couple weeks. They had one spot that we could use for a day or two, but no longer than that. We figured if we stayed a couple days there, another spot would open up, or the marina would find somewhere else for us, so we moved the boat into a tight slip between a concrete wall and a big motorboat.

Anxious to get off the boat, we went for a walk. It was an ultra touristy area with loads of restaurants and boats lined up to take people out for a one-hour tour of the waterfront. We sat down for a well-earned cheeseburger and beer, and watched the lobster colored tourists take their picture in front of the pirate flag after chasing dolphins around at sea.

We crashed hard that night. The Mediterranean passage had really taken a toll on us. We had a couple days with no wind, but for the most part we spent the last week tacking back and forth into a minimum of twenty-five knots, which is extremely exhausting after awhile. Needless to say we were very happy to be sleeping with the boat safely tied up in a marina.

We weren't too pleased when at six a.m. we woke to find the boat bucking wildly, straining the docklines. Overnight a swell had worked up and was making its way into the marina. I don't know if they just screwed up with the design of the breakwall here or what, but we had never seen anything like this before.

Monohulls were rocking and rolling in sixty degree arcs, boats were bouncing off of each other, and we were slamming off a concrete wall. Soon we had seven docklines going in every direction, many of them doubled up because they were getting chafed so badly. We also had seven fenders trying to keep *Bum* from being scraped against the wall. By eight o'clock we felt confident that we weren't going to be destroyed, but also knew there was no way we were going to spend another night in that spot.

WE GRABBED OUR MED CRUISING GUIDE and headed over to the payphone to try and find another marina. We worked our way right down the coast, having no luck. A couple of them said they had space, but as soon as I told them we were a catamaran they said no way. One place said they could give us a spot at three hundred dollars a night. We passed on that and eventually found a place in Duquesa, forty miles away and just around the corner from Gibraltar.

By ten a.m. we were underway again, and none too happy about it. Getting the boat out of our slip was a trick in itself, but somehow we managed without damage as the swell continued to roll through the marina causing havoc.

For the first hour we motored with only a ten-knot headwind to contend with. As we got further out to sea the swell flattened out and things weren't looking too bad.

I was at the nav station having a look at the charts when Ali called down to me that the wind was twenty-two knots. It had doubled in three minutes. By the time I stepped outside it was closing in on thirty and we weren't moving. With nowhere else to go we hoisted the sails and started our long tacks out to sea and back into shore again. Over and over we would perform this task throughout the day.

The wind stayed over thirty knots and we were both about ready to throw ourselves off the boat as our thirty-six mile, eight-hour trip, turned into a sixty-mile, twelve-hour bash. To top things off, we had absolutely nothing to eat. We had no fresh food left; and with our propane tank not working, we couldn't cook anything either. Eventually Ali came up with dinner, a can of tuna and a half bag of tortilla chips. At that point we had to laugh at the absurdity of the situation.

It was ten p.m. when we finally arrived in Duquesa. There was still one guy working at the marina and he helped us find our spot and tie up. It took me a few minutes to get us lined up as there was a crosswind and our spot was about twenty-three feet wide, one foot wider than the boat. Thankfully we slid right in with just a gentle bump of the fenders on our neighbor, and within minutes we were down below sound asleep.

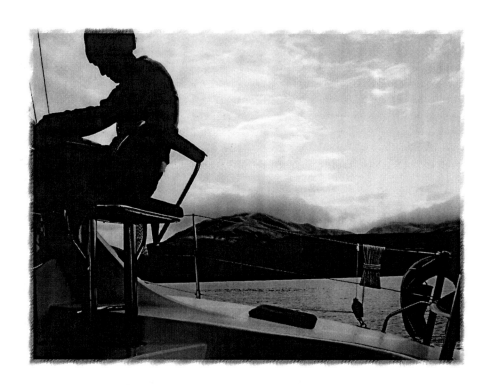

why we bother

OCTOBER 21, 2006: DUQUESA, SPAIN

After a couple weeks on land we're feeling much better about life onboard the boat again. In fact, it's sort of funny how blasé we have become about this whole sailing thing. The Atlantic crossing is coming up, and we haven't even discussed it. We know it'll be a long one, we know that we should have good weather and following trade winds, and we know we will need a lot of canned hot dogs. Aside from that what else is there to know, or talk about?

I'm sure the hundreds of cruisers lining up to head across with the ARC rally in Grand Canary would have a different take on it. But I'd also bet that at the end of the crossing most of them will say that they could have done it on their own just as easily.

Ahhh, the rallies. A couple of hundred boats lining up to take off on a specific day despite what the weather looks like, and then spending their days dodging each other while hovering for hours over their SSB radios telling everybody else where they are. God doesn't that sound like an enjoyable way to make a passage. Not exactly our cup of tea, but hey, whatever works.

OCTOBER 29, 2006: EN ROUTE TO CANARY ISLANDS

Our weather window looked a little sketchy for the first day, but it seemed like our only chance to get moving so we took it. We were out of the marina and on our way before the sun came up. All was good with the wind behind us at fifteen knots.

Throughout the afternoon, though, the wind kept climbing and we found ourselves surfing the waves with the wind up over thirty knots. At one point I saw our speed hit fourteen knots, which I am pretty sure is a record for *Bum*. We had the main double reefed and no jib out. One really nice thing about this boat is that no matter what downwind sail combination we throw up, she sails straight as an arrow.

In the afternoon I was outside having a look around when I saw that one of our two forward bimini supports had completely broken off at the weld. We'd had that same weld fixed twice previously so it probably shouldn't have been a total shock, but it was a little disconcerting considering we had over five hundred miles to go and could no longer use our mainsail.

The main is attached to the traveler which slides along the back of the bimini support, putting a lot of strain on it. With only one forward support left we couldn't take the chance of the other one breaking off as well, which would most likely result in the entire thing ripping off of the boat. So now sailing with just the jib, we continued on through the night until the wind eventually calmed down, giving us a nice motorsail towards the Canaries.

By evening of day two the wind was down to five knots and everything was quiet as Ali went to bed. Fifteen minutes later I watched the wind suddenly shift forward onto the nose and increase to fifteen knots. I called Ali up and we quickly got the screecher rolled in. Just in time too, as the wind took off to thirty-five knots.

For the next hour we bashed along wondering what the hell happened to our nice quiet night of sleep. But then as quickly as it had shown up it was gone. Just a couple of hours later we were sailing along with the screecher and a nice gentle breeze from behind.

I was asleep when Ali yelled down for me to come quick. I ran outside to find the screecher sail dragging alongside of us in the water. Ali had been sitting outside watching a nearby ship when suddenly the sail broke loose. We cut the engine, since we had been motorsailing at the time, and dragged the sail back aboard.

It was a good thing that the wind had been strong enough to launch the top of the sail away from the boat and into the water, because the top piece that connects the sail to the halyard is heavy and would have taken a nice chunk out of the topside if it had fallen straight down. It was too dark to see what had happened for sure but it would seem that once again our halyard had chafed through. So now, with four hundred miles to go, we have no main and no screecher.

Today, day three, we have virtually no wind, so the lack of sail choices isn't making much difference. A nice thing about this passage is that we have enough fuel to motor the entire way, and it's looking more and more likely we might just have to. We keep telling ourselves that it's better to have all of these things happen now rather than in the middle of the Atlantic.

NOVEMBER 2, 2006: LANZAROTE, CANARY ISLANDS

The Canary Islands passage is over. Aside from our problems with the sails there really wasn't anything to talk about. The engines worked fine as they throbbed away, one after the other, for the entire trip. There was barely any wind, making the lack of sails sort of a non issue. Dolphins visited us one time, the dinghy stayed inflated, and we ate chili dogs. It was much more reminiscent of past passages, before the Mediterranean crossing.

NOVEMBER 4, 2006: LANZAROTE, CANARY ISLANDS

"Oh, you guys are hurrying. We've been out twelve years." It had been over two months since we heard those words, leading us to believe that perhaps it had ceased being the cruiser catchphrase. But there it was again, redeeming our faith in the competitiveness of long distance cruisers.

When somebody says they've been cruising for twelve years, does it really count if they spend every winter back at their land home in the U.S.? Shouldn't that statement come with a qualification? Like maybe, "We've been cruising *off and on* for twelve years."

The way the rules stand now, a person could live on a boat for a year, move back to land for five years, then come back to the boat and say they've been cruising for six years. If it is going to be a competition then there really should be a governing body in charge of rulings on these things.

WE HAD ARRIVED IN THE CANARIES *with high hopes for surfing and sunning on the beaches. Unfortunately the weather didn't cooperate with us. We had strong wind and no swell for nearly two weeks. The upside to this was that we knocked off a lot of boat work, replacing fuel pumps, propane fittings, and having our bimini welded for the umpteenth time. When the time finally came to leave, we were grateful because it meant we could stop working.*

NOVEMBER 18, 2006: EN ROUTE TO TENERIFE

We left yesterday morning in dead calm waters, our favorite sailing weather. We puttered along the coast for a few hours and then headed out to sea for the 140 mile overnight crossing to Tenerife.

During the day we had one squall come ripping over us. There was only one dark cloud in the sky and we watched it come from miles away. By this time we were sailing, and for a minute I debated dropping the main before the storm hit. However we could see another sailboat that was right in the middle of it, coming from the other direction, and he had full sails up. Within seconds the wind went from ten to thirty knots with freezing cold rain blowing sideways through the cockpit. *Bum* galloped through the short waves, and within a couple of minutes came out the backside.

Around dark, despite the forecasts for nice gentle breezes from behind, we found ourselves getting bounced around in rough seas and thirty-knot winds. It's always disappointing when we only have a one-day passage and we find ourselves in crap weather. This time it stuck around until early morning when it gradually died down and left us to a nice cruise the rest of the way in.

NOVEMBER 19, 2006: TENERIFE, CANARY ISLANDS

With nothing to do today, and visibility down to a hundred yards due to strong winds and African dust storms, we walked up to the grocery store to buy a few more things for the Atlantic crossing.

I don't know why we bother really. We drag our feet up and down the aisles with absolutely no desire to cook any of the food on the shelves. In the end we find ourselves in the checkout line, like today, with nothing but candy bars, lollipops, bags of chips, and chocolate donuts.

While waiting in line, there was a young boy in front of us. He was about five years old and stood staring at us. At first I thought it was because of our language, but then realized he was just staring in amazement at all the good stuff we were buying. I wished I could just rustle the little guy's hair and tell him that someday when he was a grownup, he could buy whatever he wanted too. But my *Spanglish* wasn't that good, so I just gave him a smug smile and nod instead.

NOVEMBER 25, 2006: TENERIFE, CANARY ISLANDS

A few nights ago we went out to Thanksgiving dinner with a group of cruisers. Not one other person was under sixty years old, and it really highlighted for us just how different our cruising experience is from most others out here. Don't get me wrong, everybody was very nice and welcoming to both of us, but they've all got kids older than us. It's too bad everyone waits until old age to go sailing.

One thing that struck us about the conversation at dinner was how everybody wanted to make fun of the ARC. The ARC is a cruiser rally in which a couple hundred boats band together to make the Atlantic crossing, sharing weather information and helping each other out if needed. It seems unnecessary to Ali and me, and we wouldn't do it because we feel we would lose the sense of independence and adventure, but I can see how certain people would feel safer about crossing an ocean as part of a big group.

However it seemed like everyone who was making fun of the rally, was really just jealous. In fact they sat and talked about how they were going to leave the day after the ARC and listen in on the participants' radio nets. Their only problem was that so far they had been unable to obtain the radio frequencies or report times, and there were long discussions about who they could coerce into giving these to them.

Another thing we found interesting was that each of these boats had taken on at least one, and sometimes two or three crew for the crossing. And they were all busy setting up their own radio net. It sounded just like they were organizing a mini ARC, except without the big party at the end.

All of this ARC talk of course led to conversations about the weather. Cruising weather, ad nauseum. For hours and hours the talk centered on some guy named Herb whom they all use to give them weather forecasts every time they go anywhere, even in the trade winds. This Herb guy seems to take a lot of abuse for somebody who is just doing these cruisers a favor.

They bitched about him endlessly but still hung on his every word. When Ali and I pointed out that we just use GRIB files for our weather, we were treated to a long discussion about just how inaccurate this method is. I explained that it is all we have ever used and we hadn't run into any truly bad weather on our entire trip. But then our food came, and with it the end of the weather conversation.

THE NEXT MORNING WE WERE UP EARLY to run our errands. Return the rental car, pay the marina, clear out with the police, wash the boat, make sure the dinghy wasn't leaking, and do laundry.

Later on Ali was out on deck when one of the guys from dinner the other night came by to wish us well. He asked if we had gotten all of our provisioning done.

"Yeah, we grabbed a couple of bags at the grocery store the other day," she answered.

"Oh, you don't do menus?"

"Menus? Uh, no."

"So you just sort of look at the food you've got and say, 'Well that should be about right for three weeks,' then?"

"Pretty much. In a bind there is always Ramen noodles right?"

To that he just smiled, shook his head, and before walking off said, "You guys sure have a unique way of cruising."

Wait a second, is that a compliment, or . . .

A little later another couple came over to say goodbye. They weren't leaving for two more days and the lady told Ali that she had started cooking and freezing their meals a few days earlier. "Oh just twenty meals or so, to get us through the first week."

Twenty meals would get us to the Caribbean Ali thought, before saying, "Oh, that's a good idea."

This cooking thing is serious business to cruisers. I wonder if it is because so many cruisers have starved to death while crossing the Atlantic. I'll have to look that up. Actually the issue may have more to do with being in a monohull instead of a catamaran. Apparently they worry a lot more about cooking than we do because if the seas are rough it is too hard to cook with their boat heeled way over. Or maybe it's not that, maybe they just really like to eat. I don't know.

I have this image in my head of sitting at the table perusing a menu while Ali stands next to me holding a notepad and tapping her foot impatiently. "Um, I think I'll have the chili dog. Or maybe the spaghetti. No wait, the tuna fish sandwich please. What's that? Rippled or plain? Hmm, I think I'll have the rippled potato chips, please. Thank you."

IT'S NOW THE NEXT MORNING, our day of departure. Actually we're not going anywhere. The wind kicked up overnight and we woke this morning to thirty knots. We're not in that big a hurry to get moving, though now we have absolutely nothing left to do today.

Wait, strike that last comment. Ali is busy right now. She decided she was going to make herself a hard boiled egg for breakfast. She'd never done this before but it seemed simple enough. Boil water, plop an egg in, and wait a few minutes. She popped the first one in and it actually went "POP." It broke and oozed all over the place. She tried again and again. POP, POP, POP. She just gave up, defeated, and eggless. Come to think of it this may be the reason why we don't have menus and pre-made meals on *Bum*.

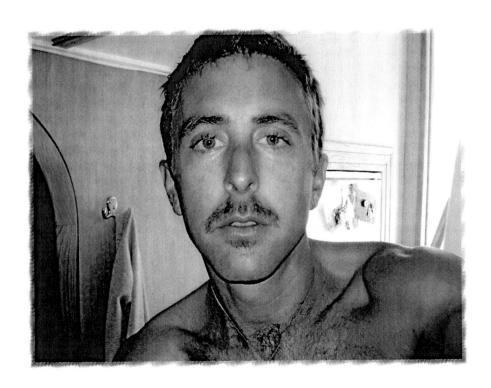

NOVEMBER 27, 2006: ATLANTIC OCEAN CROSSING

We are on our way. The last major passage of our journey and it is a pretty exciting time. I can't wait to reach the Caribbean, look at the map, and see that line across the Atlantic behind us. Ali isn't quite as excited as I am about the passage; but she is certainly in high spirits, which is pretty good for a woman about to spend three weeks at sea with nobody to talk to but me.

We definitely made the right decision not to leave the other day when the wind was howling. Instead we woke up yesterday morning and, still in the dark, slipped the lines and motored away from the dock in calm water. For about two hours we cruised along the coast before the wind came up, along with the sun. We pulled the screecher out and settled down to enjoy the best day of sailing weather we have had in at least six months.

However this morning our wind disappeared and we are left motoring again. The forecast shows nothing but good sailing weather for a few days so we're sure it will fill in soon.

NOVEMBER 28, 2006: ATLANTIC OCEAN CROSSING

On our second day out with overcast skies, the wind kept appearing and disappearing. We spent twenty-four hours motorsailing for thirty minutes, then sailing for thirty minutes.

During my two a.m. watch I was standing outside as a ship passed behind us, disappearing into the distance. Then suddenly a light popped up in front of us. While trying to figure out what it was I ran through a quick mental checklist. It was up high against the horizon, which meant one of three things. One, it was a spaceship. Not likely, since everybody knows they only fly in the desert. Two, it was a rather bright star. Mmmm, maybe. Or three, it was a sailboat with his anchor light on. That seemed unlikely since I had been standing outside and hadn't seen it earlier.

I kept looking closer, and that's when I realized that I could see the light reflecting on the water. That pretty much ruled out the star theory. They're not usually bright enough for that. A few seconds later I could just make out the white body of a boat. It was a sailboat, very close and directly in front of us.

It didn't make sense though because he was only displaying a white anchor light. No running lights. I yelled down for Ali to come up and then turned the boat thirty degrees to the right. A minute later we didn't seem to be getting any further away, and we realized that he was sailing across the front of us from left to right. We tacked over the other direction and passed just behind him. We shined our spotlight on the boat, and about thirty seconds later it shined one back at us.

In the last couple of days about 250 boats have left the Canary Islands, all headed for pretty much the same region of the globe on the other side of the Atlantic Ocean. Despite that, this guy decides to run with no lights on. Idiot. Then when he sees us he flicks on an anchor light so we can't even tell what direction he is going. That's exactly the sort of thing that Ali worries about, but that I have always told her not to because nobody is that stupid.

Today our wind filled in a bit and we had a really good day. We had a couple of accidental gybes in the morning, but once our sail setup was squared away it was nothing but smooth sailing. We've got the full main up and swung way out on one side, with half the jib out tied off to a cleat on the other side, wing-and-wing.

NOVEMBER 29, 2006: ATLANTIC OCEAN CROSSING

Into day four now and we're motorsailing again in some light fluky winds. I've calculated that we can motor about eight hours a day on average without running out of fuel. We're probably a tiny bit ahead of that at the moment; but from what I can tell, once we get a few hundred miles farther south, the trade winds should fill in more permanently and we shouldn't have any problems. That's our hope anyway.

We had another accidental gybe last night. They aren't a big deal in relatively light winds, usually just requiring us to turn on an engine and drive in a circle until we're facing the right way again. That's the easiest remedy. However this gybe set Ali off on a mini meltdown. We each go through these on long passages. Mine usually come after hanging upside down in the engine compartment for five hours thinking that I am fixing something, only to start the engine up again and find that I've accomplished nothing. Ali's meltdowns generally make her sound as if my sweet little girl has suddenly been attacked with a case of Tourette's Syndrome.

"Fuck! I fucking hate this shit! Why the fuck can't we sail this fucking boat?! What the fuck are we doing out here?! I'd rather be anywhere else than fucking here."

Usually something imaginative like that. The key for both of us is to keep quiet while the other person vents. Sometimes we do, sometimes we don't. But either way after a couple hours of sleep, the whole incident is forgotten and we are good for another week or so of carefree sailing.

We caught a couple fish today. We hadn't thrown the lines out in quite awhile, and were excited to see that we had two hooked so quickly. The first one I pulled in was a tiny mahi mahi female. I unhooked her, Ali said, "Awww, she's cute. It's okay baby," and then I threw her back in. I pulled up the other line and it was her male companion, also tiny. I unhooked him, Ali said, "Awww, he's pretty. It's okay baby," and I threw him back in. It was either that or keep them as pets.

Those mahi mahi are incredible. Popular wisdom says they mate for life. Apparently scientists disagree, but it seems that nine times out of ten when we catch them, it's in a pair. It's almost so cute that we want to join PETA and stop fishing all together. But then we remember how good they taste and get past that idea.

NOVEMBER 30, 2006: ATLANTIC OCEAN CROSSING

You know the movie *Duel*, about the guy driving his car through the desert while being harassed by a big semi for hundreds of miles? We've got the 2006 version of that movie all worked out now.

One night we're out sailing along in the middle of the Atlantic Ocean when a boat suddenly appears and cuts right in front of us with no running lights on. He freaks us out a little but then continues off to the horizon.

Two nights later we are having a beautiful night of sailing with just the screecher out in twelve knots of wind from behind. Around seven p.m. we have one last look around before the sun goes down, and there is nothing but ocean in any direction.

Four hours later, Ali wakes me up to tell me there is a sailboat right behind us with no lights on. Sure enough, in just four hours a boat managed to close from somewhere over the horizon to within a couple of hundred yards of us. Ali shines a spotlight on him and he gives a quick flash back. I go back to sleep.

Now at one a.m. the wind has climbed to around twenty knots. Ali goes to bed while I sit up to watch the sailboat that hasn't moved from his spot behind us. Seems a bit strange that in four hours he covered all those miles to get behind us, but then in the next three he couldn't manage to pass us.

An hour later the moon sets and the sky goes pitch black. Now I am really annoyed because this guy can see us, but we have no idea where he is, and therefore have to rely on him to avoid hitting us. I wait awhile and then flash the spotlight across the horizon behind us. I get nothing in return. I do this a few more times over the next hour before he finally gives a quick flash from a bit off our port side. That's better, I think, at least now he is passing us.

Around four a.m. I see a whole bunch of lights flashing around on the dark boat before a faint red one (not a running light, which would have been green on that side) is finally left on. I switch with Ali and go to bed.

Thirty minutes pass before Ali wakes me and says they seem to be getting closer again. I have a look and tell her they must have tacked, but not to worry about it. I try to call them on the VHF but they haven't answered all night. Fifteen minutes later she calls me outside again in a panic and shines the spotlight to show me why. The boat is just fifty yards in front of us now, and angling slowly across our bow. We light the boat up and yell for them to turn a light on and to get the hell away from us. I then turn us twenty degrees to the left to tack away from them.

Two minutes later Ali is standing on the other side of the boat screaming. The other boat has done a one-eighty and is now charging straight at us. At the last second I crank the boat hard over to the right as they pass across our bow a mere fifty feet in front of us. It's absolutely insane. We are five hundred miles from shore in the Atlantic Ocean and are struggling to avoid hitting some maniac in an unlit boat. When I cranked the boat to the right we spun around up into the wind and were just sort of sitting still. The other boat had done the same as they passed us and were now sitting alongside of us just thirty yards away.

We were finally able to have a good look at the boat. It was flying a French flag and looked like a normal cruising boat, about forty-five feet long, though we couldn't see a name on it. In the cockpit there was one guy at the wheel and another guy scrambling around. At this point Ali and I were both absolutely screaming at them as they just stared at us, not saying a word. If we had been in cars on the highway, this is the point I would have been dragging them out through the car window and beating them senseless on the side of the road. Fortunately, I guess, we were on boats, so instead we turned on our engines, spun around, and took off as quickly as we could.

The other boat then did the same, and also turned on all of their lights. The boat lit up, which ruled out our earlier thought that maybe they had lost all of their power in a lightning strike or something. We were both galloping through the waves at six knots, with them just a hundred yards or so behind us. Then just like that they went dark again. Our radar, which is really only useful for spotting ships, wasn't picking them up either. We altered course a bit and kept the motor on to try and put some distance between us. It was now five a.m.

A little after six the sun finally started to rise. We couldn't see the other boat, so I went back to bed. As the sky continued to brighten Ali spotted them, and again they were right behind us, a mile back. This time we'd had enough and just wanted to get as far away from them as we could. We tacked way off course and cruised along for an hour and a half at a ninety degree angle to them. They kept their course and were soon out of sight.

That was easily the most bizarre incident we have ever had out at sea. At this point, neither one of us can comprehend any possible reason for what happened. Our first thought had been that they were just idiots who didn't think it was a big deal to cross that close to another boat in the dark, unlit, far out at sea. If so, and if they don't understand English, then maybe they thought we were yelling for help or something. But if they had been coming back to help us, I don't think they would have come roaring back across our bow, cutting us off under full sails. So that doesn't make much sense. Aside from that, we've really got no idea.

For the movie script, we thought maybe they would just keep doing this sort of thing every night for a couple of weeks, depriving us of sleep until we went completely insane and jumped off the boat together, where a school of hungry sharks would quickly devour us. Something like that.

Seriously though, if these guys come back again tonight we're going to have a big problem.

DECEMBER 2, 2006: ATLANTIC OCEAN CROSSING
It's been somewhere around a week now and everything continues to go pretty well. We didn't have any repeat showing from the crazy Frenchmen, although two nights later, we did see another sailboat about a mile or two in front of us that, when it got dark, didn't turn on any running lights. We haven't had much experience with seeing other cruising boats while out at sea, so this has come as quite a shock to us. We had no idea that so many boats ran dark at night. The concept seems utterly ridiculous to us, especially on this passage with the large number of boats all sailing more or less along the same line.

We had another accidental gybe. This one broke our topping lift, the line that runs from the top of the mast to the end of the boom. Fortunately the sail itself kept the boom from falling down on top of our solar panels. We have a preventer that keeps the boom from swinging across in a gybe, but the sail itself still flops over with a lot of force which is what snapped the line.

The only repair we could come up with for now is using the spare halyard to hold up the boom. The problem with this set up is the spare halyard exits the front of the mast a few feet below the top. Everything works fine except for the fact that we can't raise the sail beyond the second reef. Fortunately with the wind currently between twenty and thirty knots, it doesn't really matter since we would be sailing with a reef in anyway.

The five-day forecast doesn't show the wind letting up, so it looks like we will just continue on like this. When and if things do calm down, I'll have Ali hoist me up the mast where I can grab the remaining half of the line which has wrapped itself around the staysail. Once I have that, I should be able to tie on an extension as a temporary repair until we get to the Caribbean.

So for now we're happily cruising along at over five knots. We tend to be pretty conservative sailors I think, which has caused us to sail quite a bit slower than we would if we pushed the boat a little harder. But we feel more comfortable this way, and really, what is another two or three days on a passage like this?

DECEMBER 6, 2006: ATLANTIC OCEAN CROSSING
The last few days we have had true trade wind sailing. The trade winds are much stronger than we expected, and they are certainly consistent. For three days we didn't touch a thing and the boat sailed straight for the Caribbean. Because of the problem with the topping lift, we have had the main double reefed the entire time, so it's kind of a good thing the winds stayed strong.

When the wind did die down for a few hours, to under twenty knots, we started looking for alternatives. We managed to re-rig our spare halyard to the other side of the mast which allowed us to raise the main all the way up, as long as it was out on the starboard side. I considered going up the mast to do a proper repair but decided that the seas were just too rough. In an emergency I could have gone up, but for this it wasn't worth the risk.

Of course once we were finally able to raise the main all the way up, the wind fired up and we had to drop it back down to put a reef in anyway. Last night the wind rose to thirty-five knots and we were surfing some pretty big waves. At one point our speed hit 14.5 knots. That was with two reefs in. After that we dropped it down to the third reef which leaves a mainsail about the size of a bed sheet, along with a handkerchief of a jib. This morning we are continuing on like that despite the slightly lower winds. Just 1500 miles to go.

DECEMBER 7, 2006: ATLANTIC OCEAN CROSSING
Day eleven, I believe, and it looks as if we will hit the halfway point today. We are really way the hell out here in the middle of nowhere now.

We received an e-mail yesterday about an ARC boat for which a MAYDAY went out. The article said that the crew called for help because they were concerned for the skipper's mental health. That's just a fancy way of saying that the skipper went crazy.

I'm not always the most sensitive guy, so normally I would get a good chuckle out of that. But having been out here on these long ocean passages I can sympathize with this nutcase. Sometimes the isolation is maddening and you just really wish you could be anywhere else in the world. Similar to being locked up in jail I suppose. Not that I would compare sailing across oceans with being locked up, but I think a lot of people, after having made a long ocean passage, could probably see the similarities.

Anyway, somebody came to the rescue, took the skipper and both of the crew members off, and abandoned the boat at sea. All they did was leave a light on. According to maritime law, that boat is now up for grabs.

DECEMBER 9, 2006: ATLANTIC OCEAN CROSSING

The past couple of days have passed with more of the same strong winds. It never seems to change out here, which I suppose is the purpose of sailing in the trade winds. We have pretty much left the sails alone the last twelve days, with only the occasional change between reef points. At night we almost always throw in another reef. If nothing else, it helps relax the person who is trying to sleep.

This morning we were sailing with one reef in the main, but we were feeling sort of silly since the wind was under twenty knots. We figured most sailors would be flying with full sails out and loving it, so we decided to pull ours all the way up too. After about an hour of this I went out to Ali, who was sitting at the helm carefully watching the wind, and said, "I know I'm a sissy sailor but I think we should put the reef back in." She enthusiastically agreed. With the reef back in we both went inside, neither of us needing to worry about an accidental gybe anymore. Maybe we're too conservative for our own good, but we always feel more comfortable being underpowered versus overpowered.

Later on I saw a boat a half-mile away just bobbing sideways in the rough seas. It seemed pretty obvious something was wrong, so I gave them a call on the VHF. Secretly I was hoping that nobody would answer and that I had just stumbled across that abandoned boat, but they answered right away. Damn. Turned out they had broken some rigging and were now awaiting the arrival of some supplies from a ship that the ARC people had routed to them. We didn't envy them as we sailed past.

At the moment, the forecast is calling for decreasing winds beginning tomorrow. Despite wanting to get the passage over with, we are looking forward to a break from the strong winds that we have had for nearly two weeks now. It's amazing how exhausting the noise of the wind and the breaking waves can be. Flatter seas, and maybe even a sail change to the screecher, would be a welcome relief right now.

DECEMBER 10, 2006: ATLANTIC OCEAN CROSSING

With under a thousand miles to go, we can let the countdown begin. Today was the kind of beautiful day that most people probably envision when they daydream about their own cruising. Fifteen knots, beam reach with the screecher sail, blue skies with puffy clouds, and just a hint of whitecap on the top of the waves. If only they were all like this. Or hell, even one a month would be nice.

DECEMBER 13, 2006: ATLANTIC OCEAN CROSSING

The happy days cannot last forever. Yesterday the wind disappeared on us. When I went to fire up the engine, I turned the key and got nothing. I had noticed the last time it started that it had been a slow crank, but figured after a few hours of charging it would be fine. I figured wrong.

We spent the rest of the day jumping and charging batteries. Not the easiest project without jumper cables. I had small chunks of wire running all over the place to make it work. Upon closer inspection, we found that the starter batteries weren't being charged at all. Somewhere in the extremely confusing mess of wiring between the alternators, starter batteries, house batteries, and regulator, there is something wrong. I'm sure to have that figured out in no time at all.

Last night we were motoring with the screecher out, more for the visual effect than anything else. There was just a whisper of a wind, but occasionally the sail seemed to give us a tiny boost. At one point I went outside to find the sail hanging limp and the wind at a whopping one knot. I went back to reading my book inside, and to wait for my turn to go back to bed.

Within less than a minute I could sense something had changed. I went outside and found the screecher backed with the wind suddenly up on our nose and rising. I tried to quickly roll it in, but the wind had already picked up to over twenty knots and the sail was flaying wildly. I yelled down to Ali, and together we tried to get the sail tacked over to the other side of the boat where we figured we could at least sail downwind and ride it out. But in the midst of all the flapping the lines had gotten tangled and we couldn't get the sail across.

In a last ditch effort, we started to drop the entire sail down onto the trampoline. We had it halfway down and piled up when suddenly I heard "RIPPP!" Then again, and again. The sail was shredding in my hands, and in seconds it was garbage. We unhooked it from the front of the boat, wrapped it in a big ball and threw it in the cockpit.

Now, with the wind really howling, we rolled out the jib and raised the main. But something was wrong with the main. That remaining piece of line from the topping lift had now managed to get stuck on the sail track and was keeping us from raising the main beyond the second reef. As a torrential downpour descended on us, we left things the way they were and huddled inside to stay dry. Why these things always have to happen at three a.m. I'll never know.

It was only a month ago that I mentioned we had never had a problem with blowing out a sail, whereas it seemed everybody we talked to and everything we read made it seem like such a common occurrence. I guess we brought this bad mojo on ourselves.

After a couple hours of the heaviest rain either of us have ever seen, the wind once again did a disappearing act and we spent the rest of the morning motoring. By the time the sun came up, the seas had gone flat. We took the opportunity to have Ali raise me up the mast so I could run a new line for the topping lift. Even with just a little bit of swell running, it was a struggle to hang on and keep from being tossed around like a tetherball.

The new line was up just in time as now, amazingly, we are flying along at seven knots under full sails with a nice twelve-knot wind at our back. Now if this could just keep up for four more days we'd really be in business.

DECEMBER 15, 2006: ATLANTIC OCEAN CROSSING

A couple nights back it looked like I was going to have to make a call for the crazy chopper to come pick Ali up. I woke to find her berating our mainsail for its insubordination, clanging in the light winds. After it received a good dressing down, I adjusted a couple of things which seemed to put it back in line. At least it stopped making so much noise.

When I woke again two hours later Ali was a new woman, helped in large part by the fact that the wind had filled in a bit and we were sailing. Truth is we are both going a little nuts at this point, ready to jump down the other's throat for the slightest infraction, or perceived infraction. Fortunately we both know the real cause of these little outbursts and are able to let them slide. We are definitely ready for landfall.

The days have been beautiful with just a couple of big white puffy clouds, sunny skies, and perfect temperatures. But then as darkness rolls in, the sky changes. About an hour before sunset the cloud cover starts to build and rain squalls appear in every direction. From that point on it is just a matter of time until we get hit. There is no moon right now, so once the sun goes down it is truly pitch black and we are sailing blind.

We have been at this long enough now that we seem to have a sixth sense about the weather. Last night Ali felt a sudden drop in the temperature and woke me up. I came outside and we just managed to get the jib rolled up seconds before a squall hit. We dropped a reef in the main and rode out the short-lived thirty-knot storm that brought plenty of rain with it. Night watches, needless to say, have been a bit of a pain in the ass.

At the moment we've got a steady breeze from behind and are flying along nicely with nothing but the main out. We're pretty excited about it since we really need to average about six knots over this last four hundred miles in order to beat our families to Grenada. Somehow we didn't think the timing of this passage through very well and have left ourselves no leeway for slow sailing. Everyone arrives in four days to celebrate Christmas in the Caribbean.

DECEMBER 16, 2006: ATLANTIC OCEAN CROSSING
When Ali felt the air cool quickly last night, she woke me to help in case we needed to drop some sail when it hit. Fortunately this time the wind wasn't that strong and we were able to keep running away downwind of it. But there was no outrunning the rain.

It came down in what seemed like solid sheets of water. I actually had to tilt my head down and tuck my chin into my chest in order to take a breath; otherwise I might as well have been trying to breathe underwater. The rain hung on longer than usual, but an hour later everything was back to normal, leaving us with a nice sail for the rest of the night.

This morning we came across another boat. At first, because of the angle, it looked like there were no sails up; and I figured that it was another boat with rigging problems or better yet, an abandoned boat. But a few minutes later we heard from him on the VHF. He told us he just couldn't sail very well in this swell and wind direction. Yet another monohull that couldn't run downwind. My dreams of becoming a pirate and commandeering another boat were dashed again. Even Ali had gotten excited over the thought of the two of us sailing single-handed side by side into the Caribbean with our new found booty.

IT'S BEEN A STRUGGLE to keep ourselves entertained these past three weeks. In our efforts, we've littered the ocean with messages in bottles and I've grown a moustache. I figured that I couldn't really be considered a salty dog without a handlebar mustache. Plus, it makes Ali laugh all day long. Literally every time we make eye contact. No matter though, I'm certain I appear much more Captainly. Of course, this thing will never step foot on land.

DECEMBER 18, 2006: ATLANTIC OCEAN CROSSING

Our last day of sailing before Grenada, after twenty-two days and 2800 miles, and it has easily been the nicest of the entire trip. The best sailing weather for us is when there is just a hint of whitecap on the waves and the swell is gently rolling up from directly behind us. That's what we had today. Combine that with a strong current pushing us along, and we are now looking at an early morning arrival.

Overall this has been about the easiest passage imaginable. For twenty-two days the only time the wind veered away from within thirty degrees of square on the stern was during a couple of short-lived squalls. In fact, if it hadn't been for us getting caught with the screecher out in one of them we could have called this a perfect passage.

Sometimes it's hard for us to imagine where the writers of sailing books find all of their drama. Maybe they make it all up. It has to be better than writing, "Today I finished another book, played Yahtzee, and took a nap in the sun. Tomorrow I plan to start a new book, play Gin Rummy, and take a nap on the couch." Which is essentially what I've just done.

DECEMBER 19, 2006: ST. GEORGES, GRENADA

A little after midnight we pulled up outside of Prickly Bay. It looked like a pretty straightforward entrance on the charts, so we hadn't really thought anything of showing up in the middle of the night. We inched our way slowly into the bay, but when I shined the spotlight around, I began seeing buoys that weren't on our charts.

We had no idea what they were for and didn't think running the boat onto a reef at this point would be a very cool thing to do, so we turned back outside the bay and anchored away from any hazards. Then at first light we pulled into the bay to find the customs man and get ourselves cleared in.

Prickly Bay was filled to the brim with boats, which I have to admit is exactly the nightmarish picture I've had in my mind of the Caribbean for the past couple of years. We have gotten a ton of e-mails telling us all about the great places to see down here, but we have kind of taken them with a grain of salt, not really sure if this would be our sort of place. A packed anchorage with nothing but cruisers swarming all over town isn't really our scene.

However after just a few minutes onshore I changed my mind. Grenada is perfectly Caribbean. The customs office was inside a pink house with plenty of purple and yellow thrown in to liven it up. There was a cute little thatched roof beach bar with a couple of locals already helping to support it at this early hour and an outboard repair shack next door with kids out front getting their makeshift fishing poles ready for the day.

The customs and immigration guys were extremely nice. I sat back listening to reggae Christmas music until our paperwork was complete. With that done we moved to the next bay over where we were meeting our families.

Just four hours later, Ali and I were sitting at the bar when their taxi arrived. How's that for timing?

IT WAS ALWAYS FUN having family visit. From them we always received a bit of perspective. They were all one hundred percent, whole heartedly, non-sailors. Aside from a couple of day sails with us, not one of them had ever spent an hour aboard a sailboat. So despite the fact that we had just endured twenty-three days sailing across an ocean in a small boat, we were immediately met by each and every one of them with, "Oh my God, that was the longest flight ever. I'm exhausted. You know we had to leave the house at seven this morning?" Ali and I would smile gamely and tell them to meet us for drinks after they were rested up.

Anybody who has ever spent a day on a boat can imagine what it must be like to spend three or four weeks at sea. But a non-sailor, including the two of us when we first set out, has no comprehension at all. And really, why would they? They don't care. It's not as if they have any intention of ever doing the same thing themselves. So whenever we were together with family, we talked about anything and everything but sailing. This, quite frankly, was just fine by us.

Grenada was a great spot for everybody to gather for Christmas. The weather was incredible, especially for a group of Minnesotans escaping below-zero temperatures back home. And best of all for our niece and nephew, Lea and Curt, Santa even knew where the island was.

It was also Curt's sixth birthday during their visit. Ali and I wanted to get him something special that would remind him of Grenada, and we found the perfect gift one day while driving around in the hills.

A worn-out sign above a miniscule home advertised handmade steel drums. We talked with the skinny old man for a few minutes and he promised to make one for us.

A few days later we returned with the kids. The old man came outside beaming and holding his latest creation. The kids were a little unsure what to think. Here we were standing in front of a decrepit home in the hills with an old black man missing the majority of his teeth. This certainly wasn't the toy store. But then we asked if he would play us a song. That guy tapped out Happy Birthday on the steel drum so beautifully I think we were all a little stunned. In the end Curt probably would have preferred a new video game, but this was much more fun for the rest of us. And hopefully it will last a little longer.

AFTER SAYING GOODBYE to the last of our family, we finally had time to think about what we'd accomplished in the last year. It had been a big one in every sense of the word. Since our previous Christmas in Bangkok, we had visited seventeen countries and sailed 13,000 miles. Four major bodies of water had been crossed, the Indian Ocean, Red Sea, Mediterranean, and the Atlantic.

We had spent 87 nights at sea. Nearly three full months was spent on overnight passages, not to mention the other twenty or so day hops. We had covered a lot of ground, and had a lot of fun.

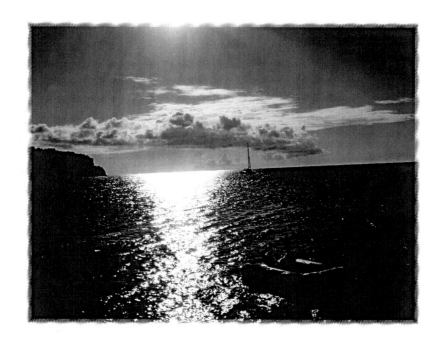

JANUARY 2, 2007: ST. GEORGES, GRENADA

For three days now, we have told ourselves we were going to move over to another nearby bay, and for three days we've done nothing but lounge around on the boat doing nothing. It seems that for the first time in quite awhile, we have absolutely nowhere to be and nothing to do. The plan is to be back in Florida in about four months. That's hardly over a thousand miles, and is practically a joke by our now skewed standards. We really aren't worrying much about anything right now, and it feels good.

Yesterday after we pulled up to the dock in our dinghy, a cruiser sitting nearby said, "Looks like a well-choreographed maneuver." It's funny how second nature certain boat-related things have become. Even seemingly simple things like pulling up to a dinghy dock. As we approach Ali stands up in front. I kill the engine and float us in, turning us right at the last moment as Ali steps off onto the dock, line in hand, a split second before the dinghy touches.

Then there are the things that give new cruisers and charterers nightmares, like docking, anchoring, and picking up a mooring. Things we haven't given even a passing thought to in the past couple of years, as they have become so ingrained and automatic. Man, we might even be able to pass one of those Captain's tests given at a local sailing school. Well, probably not. I'm getting carried away now.

JANUARY 3, 2007: GRENADA

We finally got off our lazy butts yesterday and moved. The wind was howling, but as we were only going out one bay and into the next, it was no big deal. In fact the entire move took us about twenty minutes. We're not exactly covering a lot of ground at the moment.

We moved back over to Prickly Bay for two reasons. One, we needed to go to the chandlery located there. And two, we wanted to have a beer at the beach bar. Big goals. Over the course of a couple of days we've managed to complete them both.

I must admit the chandlery took us a little longer to get around to than the beach bar. However it was unlike anything we have seen since Fort Lauderdale and West Marine. The place was stocked with absolutely every item a person could possibly need on a boat.

We wandered around for at least an hour just looking at the shelves of things that we could have used over the past couple of years. Oh the time and hassle we could have saved ourselves with just two or three of these stores spaced out around the world. Though when it came down to it, we talked ourselves out of making at least half a dozen small purchases with the simple argument that if we made it this long without them, they really must not be very important.

JANUARY 7, 2007: CARRIACOU, GRENADA

After a quick sail between the islands we arrived in Tyrrel Bay, where we found one hundred boats bobbing up and down at anchor. It's become abundantly clear that we are going to have to change our attitude about busy anchorages if we are going to have any hope of enjoying ourselves in the Caribbean.

I can count on one hand how many bays we've been in over the course of this trip that have been this busy, including places like Sydney Harbour. The constant movement of boats so close together has given us a new kind of anxiety that we aren't used to dealing with. We may have finally hit upon the reason cruisers drink so much red wine.

Fortunately with the steady winds the boats manage to stay in pretty good formation. I'm sure we'll adjust quickly. Speaking of adjusting, in our first afternoon here we saw one naked woman, one man peeing off his deck in our direction, and one set of binoculars pointed our way. There is no doubt about it, we are back in the land of the invisible cruiser.

JANUARY 9, 2007: UNION ISLAND, SAINT VINCENT & THE GRENADINES

This morning we left the country and headed over to the SVGs, Saint Vincent and the Grenadines. After looking at the charts I told Ali it was a seven-mile hop and she responded, "That's pretty far." Oh how quickly our perceptions change.

Lately the winds have been consistently over twenty knots and out of the northeast, which has made all of these little passages a bit harder than they should be. Fortunately today's was only across four miles of open sea, not leaving the waves much room to build as we stayed pretty well hidden behind Union Island the whole way over.

JANUARY 12, 2007: UNION ISLAND, SAINT VINCENT & THE GRENADINES

Ali woke at four a.m. as a storm rolled in, shifting the wind out of the south and causing all sorts of problems in the anchorage. Deck lights popped on all over the bay.

Boats that had anchored right up next to the reef were now hitting it, scrambling around frantically trying to get their anchor up. The eighty-foot catamaran behind us was pressed up against his thirty-foot monohull neighbor and putting out fenders as big as the boat to keep them apart. Meanwhile we were swinging seriously close to the charter boat that had come in and anchored five minutes before dark. Within an hour the storm passed, the typical winds returned, and the lights turned back off.

In the morning Ali and I climbed Fort Hill which overlooks the bay and the rest of the island. From the top we could see Grenada to the south and all of the Grenadines to the north. We could even scout out our next anchorage, all of four miles away, the Tobago Cays.

The wind has really been whipping the last couple of weeks, and it finally took its toll on the boat. I was sitting on the back chair yesterday when I noticed our beautiful gray MOB pole was leaning a little more than usual. Our U.S. flag at the top was really flapping and the pole was bent at a thirty degree angle. I popped it out of the holders and found that it had a big crack in it. After a quick brainstorming session with

Ali over the merits of duct tape versus hose clamps, I opted for the hose clamp fix. It worked like a charm. Though there is some doubt now as to whether or not it will still float.

JANUARY 23, 2007: ST. PIERRE, MARTINIQUE

We circled around St. Pierre for a while looking for a decent spot, but there were close to fifty boats packed into a thirty-boat area, and it was a mess. Ali took a closer look at the charts and didn't see any reason why we couldn't anchor anywhere along the coast. This particular anchorage right in front of town is the only one listed in the Doyle cruising guide that every single boat down here carries onboard, which is why nobody had anchored anywhere else.

We left the pack and motored about five hundred yards further along the island. It wasn't looking good at first as the water was still over two hundred feet deep right up close to shore, but then the bottom suddenly shot up and leveled out at just thirty feet. We circled around and found that the area was large enough for a couple of boats but we had it all to ourselves. Pure genius.

As we watched more and more boats pack themselves into the other anchorage, we couldn't wait for the sun to go down before somebody spotted us.

JANUARY 24, 2007: ST. PIERRE, MARTINIQUE

Tonight our perfect little anchorage was invaded. We knew we wouldn't be left alone for a second night, not once all the boats squished into the town anchorage noticed us looking so peaceful.

The first boat to arrive circled us a couple of times to determine if we really knew what we were doing before dropping anchor right next to us. They quickly called their friend who arrived just minutes later. Still more sheep, I mean boats, came in, and by dark we found ourselves in yet another overcrowded Caribbean anchorage. It's really becoming annoying.

JANUARY 28, 2007: PORTSMOUTH, DOMINICA

Today we set out for the quick trip to Guadeloupe. However, first we had to fix something. Just when we think that maybe we've got all of this boat stuff figured out, we do something so stupid it seems as if we have just moved aboard.

We noticed recently that our anchor chain was really twisted up. This caused the windlass to work harder and the anchor to spin in circles as we dropped it, leaving us not knowing which direction the anchor was laying on the ocean floor. I came up with a brilliant solution to the problem, though. Since we were in a deep protected bay with flat waters, we could motor to where it was 300 feet deep and drop the chain all the way out. Once it was all hanging freely it would untwist itself and we would bring it back in. Simple enough, right?

Well it turns out there was a flaw in my plan, a rather obvious one in retrospect. The flaw, 250 feet of chain is damn heavy. We removed the anchor, fortunately, and dropped the chain down. Once we reached the end, and it had untwisted, I sat down alongside the chain and got ready to pull it in. I knew it was going to be heavy, but had figured that with me pulling and the windlass cranking, it wouldn't be a big deal. Yeah, I was wrong about that.

The windlass couldn't budge it, and even with my feet planted firmly, pulling with all my might, I only managed to get it up about two links before dropping it again. I don't know what a foot of chain weighs, but assuming it's roughly two pounds, we now had about 500 pounds of dead weight hanging off the front of the boat.

We sat there a few minutes trying to figure out what to do. The only solution we could come up with was to simply drive the boat to shallower water, which would lighten the load. Now the trick was to not snag anything two hundred feet below us. If that happened we'd end up having to cut the chain away, losing all of it.

To add insult to injury, it began raining heavily while we were coming up with this, and we were expecting at any moment to have a squall come ripping through the bay to really cause us problems. We motored along slowly, oh so slowly, until we reached 130 feet. At that point we gave it another try and found that with me pulling as hard as I could, and the windlass churning away, we could just get the chain to inch its way up. After a few minutes the chain was back in the locker, the anchor reattached, and we were on our way to Guadeloupe. The only difference was that now we had a nice straight anchor chain. All we could do was shake our heads and laugh about that little goof.

FEBRUARY 5, 2007: ORANJESTAD, ST. EUSTATIUS

Tonight our quiet bay was invaded by some sort of rally. Fifteen boats from The Moorings filled with six men apiece came roaring in all at once, dropping anchors all over the field of free moorings. One boat inched alongside us and was just about to drop their anchor when I yelled over to the captain that we were on a mooring. He looked sort of confused and then pointed just a little farther in front of his boat, asking, "Is right there okay?"

I said, "No, we're on a mooring. You cannot anchor that close to us or we'll hit."

He still had a confused look on his face and finally said, "I'm sorry I don't understand what you mean."

I see that. "You know what, forget it. We'll put out fenders instead."

"Great. Thanks."

At least with The Moorings you can be sure they've got good insurance, right?

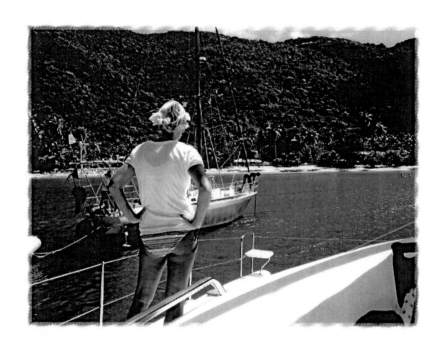

Ali's not happy

FEBRUARY 11, 2007: ANEGADA, BRITISH VIRGIN ISLANDS

It was an overnight motor to the BVIs, and with no wind it was a beautiful one. There is no better sleep than the one we get as we glide smoothly through the calm water with no noise but the quiet drone of the engine. On those nights it is hard to give up the bed when we get woken for our watch.

By morning the BVIs were in sight. And what a sight it was. The horizon was lined with white sails. A procession of them ran uninterrupted between Virgin Gorda and Anegada, our destination. For some, this is a vision they see in their dreams. For us, it is in our nightmares.

If there is one thing that we don't like about cruising, it is crowded anchorages. Ali simply does not relax or get any sleep when there are boats right next to us. She may be a bit of a worry wart, but that's just the way it is. And obviously when Ali isn't sleeping, she isn't happy. And when Ali's not happy, I'm not happy. It's a vicious circle.

But hey, we knew this coming into the BVIs, so we can't bitch about it now. Instead we just try and work around it. In Anegada that was simple. It is a flat reef island surrounded by shallow water and a few coral heads. Again, the cruising guide only lists one tiny area as an anchorage, right in front of the beach restaurants. It's a crowded area full of moorings and people trying to anchor in the midst of all of it.

There is a marked channel leading into the anchorage, where there were about fifty boats packed in, and at least another ten boats filing in behind us. While motoring through the channel, I was staring straight ahead at miles and miles of perfect pale blue waters that were completely boat free. As we came to the green buoy indicating we were to make a sharp left turn, I kept the boat pointed right where it was.

The water was seven feet deep over a fluffy sand bottom, the sun was high over our heads making any coral easy to see, and we could chose any spot over ten square miles in which to drop the anchor. Our first anchorage in the BVIs and we are all alone. Man we are good. That's the vision we should see in our dreams.

ONCE ASHORE WE SIDLED UP to a small beach bar, ordered a couple of beers, and perused the menu. After finding out how much our two beers cost, we realized there was no hope of being able to afford food. It became abundantly clear that the BVIs are for the charter crowd. For those of us accustomed to living off of beach bar food and beer this is not good.

FEBRUARY 13, 2007: TORTOLA, BRITISH VIRGIN ISLANDS

Today we packed up and sailed to Tortola. It felt as if we had joined a yacht rally. There were at least twenty boats in a tight pack all headed the same direction, with dozens more dotting the horizon all around us. This place is truly the sailing capital of the world. We have never seen anything like it before, and to be honest, I don't think either of us ever wants to again.

Our destination for the night was Guana Island. It was a pretty, relatively uncrowded bay, and after dropping the anchor I found out why. The bottom was a solid block of coral. Our anchor had just caught an edge on one chunk, but it was clear that this place wasn't going to do as an overnight anchorage. So we were off again, headed to Cane Garden Bay.

The guidebook had listed this as an excellent anchorage, so we were a bit surprised when we came in and found the entire bay crowded with moorings. There was no place left to anchor, and after nearly running aground trying to find a spot, we finally gave in and grabbed a mooring ourselves.

Cane Garden Bay is a nice enough little spot. Far from the postcard picture perfect bay the guidebook described, but nice nonetheless. There are a few beach bar restaurants lining the shore, and the beach is covered from one end to the other with beach chairs for the cruise ship passengers who visit. It has that made-for-holiday feel to it, but at night it is nice to sit on the boat and listen to the live calypso music float out over the water.

FEBRUARY 16, 2007: JOST VAN DYKE, BRITISH VIRGIN ISLANDS

The Speedo-wearing European dropped his anchor thirty feet from our mooring ball and began to back up. He then slipped back over a hundred feet before he was satisfied. We weren't.

The minute the wind changed direction he'd be wrapped around our boat. We yelled over to him that he would have to move, his boat was too close. That's when the underdressed man looked over and wagged his finger slowly back and forth at us, as if to say, Ah, you silly American children on your silly little charter boat, you know nothing.

The story didn't end there. We did convince him to move, but that's all I'm saying until the statute of limitations runs out.

The BVIs were certainly not our cup of tea. There's no doubt that it is a great place to charter a boat for a week with a bunch of friends on unlimited week-long holiday budgets. But for us, the boat crowded bays are simply too much. It is amazing just how differently cruisers and charterers can view a place. It must be the mindset of being on vacation on someone else's boat versus this being a long-term lifestyle. We heard the same thing from the other cruisers we ran into, no matter how much they hated to admit it.

FEBRUARY 18, 2007: ST. THOMAS, U.S. VIRGIN ISLANDS

We're getting to the point that we don't even like the idea of sailing for eight hours in a day. So to split the eight hour trip to the Spanish Virgin Islands in half, we stopped and spent the night on the north side of St. Thomas.

It was like a different world. Just twelve miles from Jost Van Dyke, and there wasn't another sailboat in sight. The bay was huge, over a mile deep and a half-mile across with anchoring in shallow water absolutely anywhere. It was great.

Man, I've become a recluse on this trip. Maybe we'll move to Montana, live up in the woods, and collect guns after all of this traveling. Unfortunately for that to work, our patch of woods would need to have a Taco Bell on it. Not likely.

FEBRUARY 20, 2007: ISLA CULEBRA, SPANISH VIRGIN ISLANDS
We stayed for a few days relaxing in a picturesque anchorage on Isla Culebra. It was a holiday weekend, and the speedboats from Puerto Rico filled the place each day; but by evening they all headed for home, and we were left alone, moored just feet from the beach.

Conditions changed quickly, though, and at eight this morning we had to get out of there in a hurry. Rain had shown up and the winds had shifted, bringing with it a big swell that was trapping us in the horseshoe-shaped bay. The pass through the reefs to get out wasn't complicated, but with the huge seas it was a little unnerving. The shallow coral areas were easy to see by the breaking waves, but we had to motor over a few spots that were only ten feet deep with the swell heaving and threatening at any second to begin breaking. After clearing the mile-long pass, we were out in the open and running downwind.

We made our way to Dewey on the island of Culebra and grabbed a free mooring right outside of town. As of right now it is still pouring rain and we haven't left the boat. However with absolutely nothing onboard to eat, rain or not we'll be heading in this afternoon.

FEBRUARY 23, 2007: ISLA DE VIEQUES, SPANISH VIRGIN ISLANDS
Yesterday we moved a few miles down the coast to Puerto Ferro, one of two famous bioluminescent bays on the islands of Vieques. This was a small bay with a tiny entrance as shallow as five feet in places. The water was sort of green and wasn't all that great for swimming, but we were there for the night show anyway.

We've seen bioluminescent displays hundreds of times, always while we are underway. Most often the best displays were when the prop wash would come swirling out from the back of the boat. We could watch for hours as the bright green balls of light slipped behind us. Occasionally we'd get lucky and on a really dark night be joined by dolphins that would leave perfect glowing trails of green in the darkness behind them. Anyway, the point is that we have seen the stuff, just never had the chance to swim in it ourselves.

After dark we went outside and shook the dinghy line around in the water a bit, but didn't see anything. We waited another hour and tried again, still nothing. There was a half moon out and it wasn't all that dark, so after a few hours we gave up and went to bed.

Around four o'clock I woke up and decided to go have one last look. The moon had set and it was very dark now. I lifted the line to the dinghy again, gave it a swirl, and watched as an explosion of green light came off of it. Ali came outside for a look as I jumped in for a swim. It was awesome.

I believe, but don't hold me to it, that the green lights are a defense mechanism that these microscopic organisms give off when they are disturbed. So by jumping into them it looked as if my body lit up. Underwater I could watch the lights emanate from my fingertips as I swam along. My fingers looked like the end of a magician's wand, or like the fairy dust in a cartoon movie. She won't admit it, but Ali really enjoyed watching me swim around naked with all of my extremities looking very Hulk-ish.

It was a pretty cool experience, one that can only truly be appreciated off the back of your own boat anchored in your own bay. To me this was what cruising was supposed to be about.

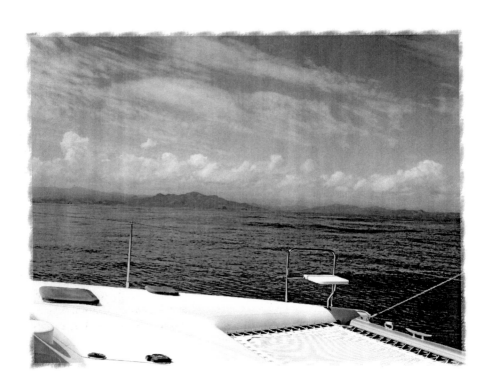

MARCH 19, 2007: PUNTA MACAO, DOMINICAN REPUBLIC

This morning at 6:30, I found Ali drinking coffee and happily typing out e-mails, actually excited to get going. So we did. The thing about these early morning starts is that by the afternoon it starts to feel like the longest day ever, especially when we are going on an overnighter. By four o'clock our early morning enthusiasm for passage making had disappeared. But with nowhere nearby to drop anchor, we didn't have much choice so we continued on into the Mona Passage.

To be honest I hadn't read about this little section of water and didn't even know it had a name, but after awhile I started to get curious about what was going on. There seemed to be at least three distinct wave directions at all times. We were encountering some of the sloppiest seas we'd ever had, and in only ten knots of wind.

I broke out the cruising guide and found that because of a number of different technical reasons, this is generally not a very fun hundred mile stretch of water. Throughout the night the boat continued to be tossed about willy-nilly, making all sorts of noise, and eventually even chafing through our reefing line. Yes, we had a reef in with just ten knots of wind. Not because of the wind though, but because we have a broken section of track at the top of the mast and we haven't been able to find the parts needed to fix it. It really wasn't that bad, though, just an uncomfortable night of bouncing around in a small sailboat.

By noon we had dropped anchor at Punta Macao, in the Dominican Republic. The aforementioned guidebook stated that we would not have seen a prettier cove since the Bahamas. That was far from true, but I suppose the author did write that thinking we would have come here straight from the Bahamas instead of the slightly roundabout way that we actually took.

Honestly though, it is a very pretty little spot with nice clear water and mile upon mile of palm-studded beach. When we arrived, the beach was deserted except for a few local fishing boats that were pulled up to the high tide line.

MARCH 21, 2007: SAMANÁ, DOMINICAN REPUBLIC

What a long twenty-four hours it has been. When we woke up yesterday morning, a swell had developed and was making its way into the bay. By the afternoon it had officially become a problem.

The bay had a nice big entrance during calm weather; but in a swell this size the northern part of the entrance, which was between six and ten feet deep over coral, was now nothing but heaving mountains of breaking white water. The southern part of the entrance was a headland which the swell wrapped around before slamming into rocks and creating more nasty breaking waves.

This left us with a very narrow and very dangerous exit between the two. Also, we were anchored in just twelve feet of water, and I was becoming concerned that if the swell grew much bigger we would suddenly find ourselves anchored on the inside of a beach break. Our plan had been to leave that night just before dark, but by three o'clock we knew we had to get out of there.

Fortunately this is one of those stories where all the drama is in the anticipation. The actual escape went flawlessly. A couple of the swells we rode out felt like they were just on the verge of building up on themselves and toppling over; but they never quite reached that point, and we slid over them easily while holding our breath.

Immediately outside the reef in sixty feet of water, everything felt better. Sometimes the safest spot to be is out in the open ocean. Just a few minutes later we were treated to a huge humpback whale spewing spray just a hundred yards in front of us, arching his back, and leaving an oil slick behind for us to drive the boat through. We have arrived right at the end of breeding season but are hoping that this won't be our last encounter with these beasts.

LAST NIGHT WAS PITCH BLACK with no moon at all. As so often seems to be the case on nights like this, something was bound to go wrong. I was on watch when the autopilot started beeping, telling me that it couldn't keep us on course. I knew immediately what the problem was. I grabbed the spotlight, shined it off the back of the boat, and saw what I'd expected. A line of fishing net buoys.

Having heard the commotion, Ali came outside and we talked over our options. Truly there weren't any options. The boat couldn't move while the net was wrapped around the prop. I needed to get in the water and cut it. In normal conditions this wouldn't be a big deal, but in the middle of the night with twenty knots of wind and a big swell there was a slight hesitation.

The biggest danger was getting separated from *Bum*. Even with no sails up the boat was still moving along at one and a half knots. We tied a couple of docklines together and I threw a loop over one arm before jumping in with my dive knife in hand. Ali was perched with the spotlight out over the edge of the boat as far as she could reach without falling in herself.

On my first dive I sliced half of the net loose. Now, with just one line around the prop and the rest of the net trailing out the other side of the boat, came the tricky part. With the line in one hand, I had to grab the prop with the other, and spin it loose with the boat riding up and down in the swell. It was a good thing I had just scraped the barnacles off the prop a couple of days earlier.

Anyway, no sharks showed up to eat me, the boat never crashed down on my head, and I didn't get caught in the net. With a little teamwork, we managed to get ourselves untangled and back underway in fifteen minutes. To be honest I was kind of glad it happened. It was sort of a man-versus-sea kind of night, which surprisingly are few and far between out here. Sometimes this sailing business can get a little tedious, and I can use the excitement.

WE ARRIVED IN SAMANÁ very early in the morning but still had visitors almost immediately. Three men arrived, one wearing some sort of official uniform, another acting as his sidekick, and a self-proclaimed translator. They came on the boat to fill out some truly ridiculous paperwork.

At one point, one of them asked me the name of our boat. Instead of saying and then spelling it, I pointed it out to him on our boat registration paperwork so he could copy it down. A minute later I saw what he wrote and had to stifle a laugh. The spot I had pointed to said Vessel Name at the top and Bumfuzzle underneath it. So what did he write for our name? Yep, VESSEL NAME.

Next, leaving Ali at the boat, the rest of us went into town to finish up with the other offices. Here in the DR "gifts" are a natural and expected way of life. I gave the two officials an unofficial two bucks each which they seemed truly pleased with. The translator wasn't letting me go though and wanted to lead me to the next office.

For a couple bucks I figured I'd go ahead and let him do his thing, so I followed him across the street. In the park we ran into his associate who, as it turns out, also deals in fine jewelry. After I declined their generous offers to view the gems they had for sale, Mr. Translator said he would send this guy to buy a DR flag for me. Once again I turned him down. This seemed to perplex him.

"There is only one store that sells them, though."

Uh huh. "Well maybe you could tell me where it is after we finish up here," I said.

Still in the park we now ran across the very man whom we were going to meet at the port authority office. What a stroke of luck. And oh, surprise surprise, he could do the paperwork right here on the park bench for me. The port authority guy whipped a receipt out of his pocket and began filling it out. These guys must have thought I was a real idiot, or that this was my first trip away from home, to think that I was falling for any of this. It was all so transparent.

I watched him fill out the receipt and then he told me the total I owed was $24.50.

I said, "Really? I thought it was supposed to be much cheaper than that."

They spoke some rapid-fire Spanish between themselves and agreed that yes, twenty dollars would be fine.

"You know what, I'd be more comfortable if we went up to the office," I told them.

A quick glance occurred between the two of them before they agreed, and we all trudged across the street.

Inside was a lovely woman who was clearly in charge of the port authority office. A few words were exchanged before the announcement that, "Ahh, there has been a mistake with the calculations. This woman here will finish the paperwork for you." And finally, after paying fifteen dollars, it was time to go see immigration.

On the way over there, my new friend slash translator, Richard, told me his fee was separate from the payments to the various offices. I rolled my eyes and asked how much. "Thirty dollars," he replied with a straight face.

It was hard not to laugh but I'd had about enough of Richard and his little scams, so I peeled off four dollars and handed it to him, telling him, "Thanks for the help but I'll take it from here."

He was none too pleased with this and let me know it. I told him that it might have been more had it not been for the ruse in the park. Now he was outraged. How could I possibly accuse him of conspiring to part me from my money in such an unsavory fashion? He went on like this for a few minutes before finally giving up and leaving me to finish my paperwork with immigration. It had been a comical morning.

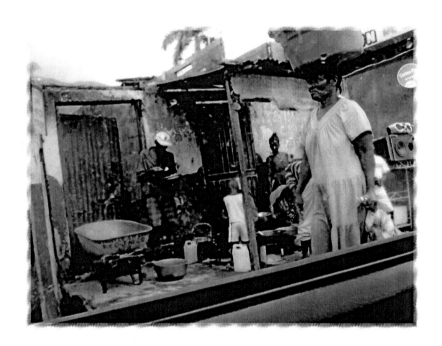

tap–tap to O'Cap

MARCH 24, 2007: LUPERÓN, DOMINICAN REPUBLIC

We didn't spend a lot time in Samaná, pretty much covering the town in just a few hours. After a couple of days we moved on to Luperón.

Our charts for Luperón showed nothing but a giant gray blob. So with just an old sketch from a guidebook, we proceeded into the mangrove-lined bay. The entrance was easy, but once inside there were mud shoals everywhere. We proceeded forward as slowly as we could, at one point just missing running aground. We quickly backed away and made our way into the anchorage.

I knew this was a popular cruiser stop, but had no idea that so many boats would call this swamp home. There were around a hundred of them in the bay, most of which looked as if they had been there for a very long time.

It didn't take long for someone to come by and let us know about the cruisers net at eight every morning. That is always a sure sign that the cruising lifers have turned a place into a retirement village.

After checking in with the authorities, we went for a walk around town. It was Saturday and everybody was out and about. We exchanged many smiles, waves, and *holas*.

For such a ramshackle town, there were a surprising number of nice restaurants, seemingly all run by expats with Dominican wives. We pulled up chairs at one which overlooked the busiest intersection in town, where dozens of *motoconchos* waited for their next customer. Everybody seemed to gather there, to say hi and discuss their plans for the weekend. There would be no big weekend plans for us, though. Like a couple of old fogies, we were home and in bed by eight o'clock. Those overnight passages wipe us out.

MARCH 28, 2007: LUPERÓN, DOMINICAN REPUBLIC

While continuing to enjoy the torrential downpours in Luperón, we decided to head to the yacht club, where two things happened to remind us yet again that we simply don't fit in with the "real" cruisers of the world.

The first incident happened while Ali and I were eating lunch overlooking the boats anchored in the harbor. An old guy proudly wearing his standard issue gray beard approached us and asked, "Do you work here?"

We both realized at that point, we had reached a new low. Not only was this guy sure that we weren't cruisers, he had also determined that we probably worked at this rundown Dominican Republic marina where employees earn somewhere quite a bit south of a buck an hour. It may be time for us to buy some new clothes.

As it turned out he was from SoCal and was considering coming here next season with his fifty-eight footer and needed some information on a berth. After we pointed out the lovely Spanish-speaking, dark-skinned girl behind the bar he seemed to decide that this wasn't the place for his yacht, and left. I guess Ali and I blend in better with the locals than we do with the cruisers.

Next we were on the internet where we found out that the chat rooms have banned *Bumfuzzle*. The cruisers forum website where I am proud to say, the *Bumfuzzle* topic holds the record for the most discussed ever, has locked all *Bumfuzzle* threads from further discussion and apparently is now even deleting new threads that mention us. The thing that gets me is that this site's tagline reads, "Discussion board and photo gallery for cruising sailors and wannabes." And here I thought that our website was a pretty good resource for those very people. Guess not, as the "real" cruisers who run the site have concluded that our story is irrelevant to those wannabe cruisers and needn't be discussed any further.

So with the evidence piling up, it appears we've failed in our quest to become real cruisers and join their mighty ranks. Perhaps we'll reach that pinnacle the next time around when we're a little older and a lot wiser. Fingers crossed.

MARCH 30, 2007: CAP-HAITIEN, HAITI

As tends to happen with us occasionally, we start to go a little stir crazy after just a day or two on the boat. We wanted to rent a motorcycle but the rain kept us from doing that, and car rental prices would have us believe we were actually in New York City. So, needing something to do, I announced to Ali we were leaving in the morning for Haiti, the western hemisphere's poorest country. It was sure to be an adventure, something that has been sorely missing in the tame Caribbean.

This morning we packed a small bag with a couple of shirts and jumped in a shared taxi. It took us a total of four taxis and buses to get to the border. At one point a bus dropped us off seemingly in the middle of nowhere and told us that the next one we wanted would be along shortly. True to their word a bus going our way came by within seconds. We hadn't waited more than two minutes between modes of transportation the whole morning on the DR side of the border.

When we arrived in Dajabón, the DR border town, it felt as if we'd landed on another planet. The streets were packed with people, and we had no idea which way to go. We figured finding a border crossing in a small town shouldn't be too complicated but nobody we asked for help had any clue what we were talking about. We eventually came across a couple of United Nations soldiers who were full of smiles and pointed us in the right direction. As soon as we were on the right street, the mass of humanity swept us along to the border.

This border crossing was like nothing we had ever experienced before. Our minds were on overload taking in all of the sights around us. It seemed as if the entire town had been turned into a market where anything and everything was for sale. Skewers of miscellaneous meat cooked over old oil drums, plastic lawn chairs were piled two stories high, women carried live chickens by the feet while balancing racks filled with dozens of eggs on their heads, boys pushed wooden-wheeled wagons full of fresh produce, and on and on.

There was a different feeling in the air as well. We saw two fist fights break out, and the laid-back, friendly DR suddenly felt like it had a much grittier edge.

This was all before we had even passed through the gates to the border crossing itself. We went up to the immigration window where we had the honor of paying $25 U.S. dollars each in order to leave their country. Nothing gets me more worked up than exit fees, and the fact that even here, on the border between the Dominican Republic and Haiti, we have to pay them in U.S. dollars.

We proceeded across the bridge over the appropriately named Massacre River. Here the police seemed angry and were using a bit of abuse in order to keep everyone moving in a single file line. We were quickly singled out and asked to produce our passports, after which we were pointed to the Haitian immigration office.

Crossing the bridge and looking at the other side was an eye-opening experience. On the Haitian side of the border were thousands of people, trucks loaded down with goods of all sorts, and mud everywhere. It had been raining for fifteen days straight and the ground had turned to soup.

The Haitian officials stamped us in easily and after exchanging some U.S. dollars for the Haitian gourde, pronounced *goo*, Ali and I jumped on a motorcycle and headed for the bus station. How a guy can steer one of these little motorcycles with three adults on it, in mud six inches deep, is beyond me. Ali was sure that at any second we were going over, but we made it to the station no problem and began asking around for a *tap-tap* to O'Cap.

This is about the time we started to feel a little uncomfortable. It wasn't as though we felt threatened, but we just weren't getting much of a reaction from the locals at all. Eventually a guy pointed us onto his bus and we climbed in. It was absolutely the scariest mode of transportation we had ever been in.

The bus was really some sort of truck with a heavy duty roof on it, just high enough to clear my head while sitting down. Inside the back were bench seats along each side and one right down the middle. We sat down on the middle bench all the way towards the front. It was clear that in an accident, there would be no escape for us. That point would be driven home once the truck had thirty bodies packed inside so tightly that we couldn't move our legs.

The menacing-looking guy who had put us on the truck, now hung in the window demanding his money. I handed him 200 *goo*, which from watching the others was a more than fair price. He made it clear that wasn't enough. The language in Haiti is Creole/French, which is simply the most complicated language ever to hit our ears. So we were more or less communicating by sign language. He said 600. I told him 200. Then get out, he told us.

Well Ali and I weren't really liking the looks of this bus depot, and we weren't about to get off a bus we knew was going to the city we wanted. We stayed put. He got angrier, and I showed him that I only had 350 *goo* total, ten dollars. Finally a girl sitting across from us tried to speak up on our behalf. The guy was having none of it, though, and demanded the 600 *goo*, which was four times the local rate. The truck was packed now and we were holding things up, so we finally gave in, exchanged more money, and settled in for the wonderful ride.

THE TRIP FROM THE BORDER to O'Cap took over two hours on horrendous roads. Signs of the roads destructive powers were everywhere, as huge trucks rotted on the roadside, most with snapped axles.

The scenery along this stretch was pretty amazing. One second we'd see a baby naked and covered in mud, the next would be a young girl wearing a pristine white dress. However, the homes were always the same, nothing but sticks rising out of the mud to form four walls.

Finally arriving in Cap-Haitien, our friendly girl from the bus helped us get a taxi. She first told us the price the driver wanted, 700 *goo* for a five minute drive, which was more than the robbery we had just endured for a two-hour bus from the border. We laughed that off and he immediately dropped his asking price by four hundred percent. We quickly learned that the people of Haiti are mighty poor, but it isn't due to a lack of trying.

By the time we checked into the hotel, which was also priced about three times too high, our system was in a state of overload. We washed away the dirt of the day with a blessedly hot shower and then washed the rest of it down with an ice cold Prestige beer at the hotel bar.

MARCH 31, 2007: CAP-HAITIEN, HAITI

I'll be honest, yesterday when we arrived at the hotel we were both a little shell shocked. Even with all of the traveling we've done, we were still unprepared for Haiti. "Seething mass of humanity" is an overused saying, but that is exactly what we found ourselves in. The filth was shocking, the living conditions were shocking, the roads were shocking, and the sheer number of people all around us was shocking. But we regrouped.

After having escaped to our hotel for a night of rest, we were ready to venture back out. We wanted to see the great sites of the Sans-Souci Palace and the Citadelle Laferrière.

The hotel receptionist was a tough nut to crack. She spoke English but would give us no information beyond answering our questions with a yes or no. After dozens of questions like this we finally determined that we could hire a taxi to drive us around for the day. It was either that or take a *tap-tap*, but we hadn't quite recovered that much from the previous day yet.

The taxi driver started our negotiations with an astronomical price. Where they come up with these numbers I cannot imagine. His first price would have put him on par with a Fortune 500 CEOs salary. The numbers tumble rather quickly though, and soon we had him down to a much more reasonable McDonald's junior manager salary, a number which, after witnessing the condition of the road and the beating his car took, we felt compelled to raise.

It was only a twelve-mile drive to Sans-Souci, but it took over an hour to negotiate the roads and the checkpoints. Watching rural life go on outside our taxi cab window was worth the trip all by itself. It felt like we had been transplanted inside a National Geographic magazine. The poverty was intense, but so were the colors, the beautiful faces of the people, and the smiles and laughter of the children.

SAN-SOUCI PALACE WAS BUILT IN 1810 to rival Versailles in France. The fall of the ruler it was built for, along with an earthquake, ruined the place within just thirty years. The palace walls still stand largely intact, however, and we got a definite feel for what it must have been like in its heyday.

The ruins were beautiful and the grounds that they sat on were incredibly picturesque. We shook off a few guides there, and then started up the hill for the Citadelle. The Citadelle Laferrière is a mountaintop fortress built to defend against the French. The guidebook said it was a three mile walk, and we knew it was perched on a mountaintop, but neither of those two facts really settled in our minds until a bit later.

For now we were content to continue saying no to the guides who asked us to ride their horses up the mountain. One look at the poor skinny creatures with open sores on their backs and we knew there was no way that we could be a part of that.

The walk up the mountain, as with everywhere else in Haiti, left us speechless. The living conditions were mere squalor, but yet again, we marveled at the people. The children were giggling, playing, and eager to say *bonjour*. The numerous women with huge buckets of laundry balanced on top of their heads were amazing.

One lady had us feeling as if we were characters in the story of the turtle and the hare. We passed her early on, only to find ourselves exhausted shortly after. We sat down for a break and watched as she steadily climbed towards us. Before she'd reach us we'd take off again. We repeated this at least half a dozen times over the next two hours. Yes, the three-mile climb actually took us two and a half hours. It was grueling, and yet at the top, there were still small homes tucked in along the path and little old ladies walking up and down as if they'd done the trip twice a day for the past seventy years. The women here are tough, no doubt about that.

We were honestly starting to wonder if we would make it to the top when the Citadelle finally came into view. It really was a marvelous sight to behold. Peeking out of the clouds high above us, we could see it framed between the banana trees.

Before we could get there we had to negotiate one last area full of very persistent guides who looked at us quizzically before asking, "Where is your guide?" Obviously they were a little stunned to see us by ourselves. The guides then tried the old Egyptian scam of getting us to hand over our tickets to them. They didn't like it too much when we just held the tickets out for them to see but wouldn't let them have them.

By this point of the climb, Ali was really hurting and probably contemplating pushing me off once we reached the top. This last stretch was a mile straight up, but upon reaching the Citadelle it was worth it. The thick walls and steep mountain cliffs make the place feel truly impenetrable. Luckily for us, the gate was open and we could wander right in.

Inside, the walls were dripping with moss, blazing green and orange. There were row upon row of two-hundred-year-old cannons, all etched with elaborate carvings, and huge piles of cannonballs still sat at the ready beside them. This fact really impressed me, because I just could not believe that a group of kids hadn't discovered the fun of launching the cannonballs over the wall and watching them smash down the mountainside. At twelve years old I would have found that irresistible, and even now had a hard time refraining.

We climbed up to the top overlooking the entire valley. If we had a clear day, the views would have been spectacular. As it was we had another gray overcast day, which did add a sort of eeriness to the place.

It had taken us close to three hours to make the climb up the mountain, and it took half as long to make the hike back down. We were long overdue by the time we reached our taxi, but our driver seemed unsurprised as we loaded in for the long drive back to the hotel.

A little extra pay at the end of the day brought big smiles to all of our faces, as Ali and I were exhausted and sore but thrilled at having just visited one of the most amazing and most inaccessible places we're ever likely to visit.

APRIL 1, 2007: CAP-HAITIEN, HAITI

By the morning of day three in Haiti we were feeling much more at ease with the country. The people would crack a smile after we spoke to them, and it became clear that their brash ways were not really meant to be as angrily abrasive as they at first came across.

With that in mind we got in a taxi for the quick trip back to the *tap-tap* station. Before we got in the car I showed the driver the 100 *goo* I would pay him for the ride and he motioned for us to get inside. Upon arrival smack dab in the middle of the bustling bus parking lot, we got out and handed him the money.

"*Non,*" he yelled.

"*Oui oui,*" I yelled back.

No, yes, no, yes. We went on like this for a couple of minutes while a large crowd gathered around us. Each new person would come up, listen to the driver's story and then show me with their fingers that yes indeed I should pay him two hundred.

Soon I had the money back in my hand and was waving it in front of his face, indicating how I had showed him the money before we left. He would yell back at me for two hundred. Ali was disappearing further and further back in the crowd, but a quick glance her way and the smile on her face told me that she was fine. In fact she was enjoying the scene as much as everybody else. She told me afterwards that a few people had indicated to her through hand gestures and smiles that it was okay.

Finally, after a good five minutes of arguing, the driver snatched the hundred *goo* out of my hand, climbed in his car, and raced off, swearing the entire time. This brought about a good deal of laughter and we were quickly shown to a bus, where we were given the same rate as the locals, one hundred *goo*. We'd earned ourselves a little respect.

THIS *TAP-TAP* WAS AN OLD SCHOOL BUS, not the speeding death truck we had ridden here in. Each seat, designed for two children, was filled with three grown adults. It was crowded but it had working windows, which made all the difference.

As the bus filled up, our third seat became the last one open. People would climb on the bus, have a look around, see our seat, and climb back off. Nobody wanted anything to do with sitting next to the white people. Eventually a young guy came on and, despite the taunts of the others around us, sat down beside me, bringing a good deal of laughter. You could see it was all in good fun, though, and before long we were underway.

The ride was torture. We couldn't imagine how an old school bus could take that sort of abuse. Two hours in, and we got our answer. The bus came to a sudden stop in the middle of the road and people began climbing out. We stayed put for a few minutes, but listening to the driver grind the gears while trying to get the transmission to engage finally drove us outside as well.

Before long the motorcycles started appearing. We weren't quite ready to give up yet, but after a half-hour of working on the bus, the driver announced that it wasn't going anywhere. Ali and I jumped on a *motoconcho* and sped off. We couldn't believe our eyes when two minutes later we were racing through the now dusty border town.

The border itself was a ghost town compared to Friday. The UN convoys, with their white SUVs and tanks, were still there in force, as they had been all over the country. But the people were gone. We cleared out of Haiti, paying another U.S. denominated exit fee in the process, and made our way across the bridge.

Back on the DR side, we went to immigration to clear in, paying yet another ten U.S. dollars each. We had traveled by public transportation and stayed in a rundown Haitian hotel for two nights, yet thanks to border fees this had become our most expensive two-day trip ever.

By now we were out of U.S. dollars. I told the officer I had none and would have to pay him in pesos. He was having none of it. I could not enter their country using their currency. After some pointless arguing, we eventually were left with no option but to exchange pesos for U.S. dollars at a ridiculous rate with a black market money changer who sat directly in front of the immigration window. With that done we were once again welcome to spend pesos freely.

Walking down the street of this dilapidated Dominican Republic border town Ali made the comment, "God is it nice to be back in civilization."

I think the average person might have felt that civilization was a strong word for where we were, but she was right. We bought a couple of Cokes and a bag of Doritos to prove it.

Somehow we managed to negotiate the four buses and taxis it took to get back to Luperón, including another bus breakdown, and we made it to the boat just minutes before darkness settled in. We had left the hotel at eight o'clock and it had been a long day, but an awesome weekend getaway.

APRIL 2, 2007: LUPERÓN, DOMINICAN REPUBLIC

Back on the boat today we could hardly move. Our legs were so sore from the mountain climb the other day that we've been popping aspirin like it is candy to try and relieve the pain. We did manage to get a few things done, though. We got our last batch of diesel, fixed a few more dinghy leaks, bought candy bars, a couple loaves of bread, and had a few beers along Main Street. With that accomplished we should be ready to take off from here soon.

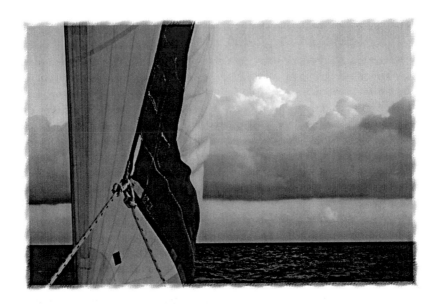

grand finale

We had heard Luperón referred to as Chicken Harbor #2, number one being George Town, Bahamas. The implication being that this is the kind of harbor that weak-kneed cruisers sail into and then never leave because they are too scared to venture any further.

Yesterday, while we were sitting at the bar we finally understood the full extent of that. The bar we were at had their VHF radio on scan, meaning it picked up all the cruiser chitchat in the harbor. During our short afternoon there we must have heard the name Chris Parker, a guy who makes a living predicting weather for Caribbean sailors, a dozen times.

"*Windancer, Windancer,* this is *Windsong.*"

"Go ahead *Windsong.*"

"Chris Parker says we have a good weather window to sail for the Bahamas."

"Roger that *Windsong.* I was speaking with *Windcatcher* earlier and he reported that Chris Parker says we should have good weather for the next few days."

"Copy that *Windancer.* So are you and Henrietta going to go for it?"

"Well I'm not sure yet, we're talking to *Windreamer* about it, but he's thinking maybe we should wait one more day. Parker says we should have winds under ten knots then."

"Roger that. I also heard *Windwalker* calling on the VHF earlier asking if there were any local boats that could lead them out of the harbor. Have they had any luck with that?"

"That's a negative, so far no luck, so we may have to stay a few more days while we have an exit channel marked."

The conversations went on in this vein for hours. It was great entertainment while sitting at the bar getting pissed. Funny thing about all of this Chris Parker talk was that I had known for five days that we'd be leaving on the 4th. I really can't understand all the discussion about weather in the Caribbean. The weather here has been the most consistent of anywhere we've been.

It blows from the northeast every single day. The only question is how hard. Will it be ten, fifteen, or twenty knots? It takes me literally ten seconds to open up the weather file that I get through e-mail, look at the little wind arrows, and determine if we are going out sailing or not. I receive a five-day forecast which is nearly always spot on. We honestly use nothing else.

So with our departure date blessed by the weather guru, I went in at eight o'clock this morning to go through the ridiculous paperwork shuffle again. The immigration officer whom I'd spoken to the day before, and who had said he would be there at eight o'clock didn't show up until nine. When done with him, I paid my harbor dues with the port authority, and then moved on to the Navy where I paid another twenty dollar fee. That last fee finally put us over the top, and DR officially became the most expensive country ever in terms of official fees.

At ten o'clock we finally inched our way out of the harbor, following our old track out, and avoiding all of the mud bars scattered throughout the place. Outside we found absolutely perfect conditions, almost no swell with a twelve-knot breeze from behind. We had a great day, even managing to catch a nice current running in our direction.

We had a strange occurrence when a group of tuna joined us and swam ten feet in front of the boat as if they were dolphins. They stayed there for half an hour before veering off.

Right now, it is the middle of the night and we've got a nearly full moon lighting up the ocean, making it a perfect night as well.

APRIL 6, 2007: EN ROUTE TO BAHAMAS

The weather remained nice for our second day out, leaving us with nothing to do but lie in the sun and count the hours until we could go to bed again.

About an hour before dark we turned the port engine on. I never got in the habit of checking the exhaust after starting an engine, but Ali always does, and she commented right away that the engine was smoking. I had a look at it, but blew it off thinking that the DR fuel we got must have had a little water in it. A few minutes passed before it dawned on me that I hadn't put any DR fuel in that tank. I went back out for another look and realized there wasn't a whole lot of water flow coming out.

We shut the engine down and it was clear right away that the engine had been running hot. I got to work and removed the old water pump impeller. It had one flipper left out of six, with three of the broken pieces still jammed in the pump. I slipped a new one in, fired up the engine, and presto; no smoke, lots of water, cool engine.

TEN MILES LATER, at eleven o'clock, we became official circumnavigators by sailing across our outbound path between the Bahamas and Panama. I suppose there should have been some sort of celebration, but I was sleeping and Ali was in the middle of a good book. We're really sentimental like that.

A short while later I was sitting outside messing with the GPS. I wanted to check what the moon would be doing for next week's passage to Florida, and the GPS has a feature that shows us the moon's position, stage, rise and set times. We always enjoy night passages more with a big full moon.

Anyway, I reached over, pushed the button, and the screen went blank. I wiggled the cord a bit but couldn't get it to come back on. I grabbed the flashlight for a closer look and found one of the four pins that make the electrical connection had fallen right off. Ali remarked later that it reminded her of those people who turn 100 years old and then die during their birthday party. I guess this GPS had had enough. It reached its milestone and then crapped out. Fortunately we had with us a young whippersnapper of a GPS just waiting to take its coveted space at the cockpit control panel.

APRIL 7, 2007: JAGGED ISLANDS, BAHAMAS

Last night we ran into one of the worst storms we have ever encountered at sea. Thankfully it only lasted about twenty minutes. The moon hadn't come out yet and the sky was black. However, we could still see the milky gray storm cloud across the horizon.

Ali woke me up before we reached this one, knowing that it was going to be a doozy. We only had the jib out as we approached it, but even that turned out to be too much when we got hit. The wind screamed from under ten knots to close to forty in a matter of seconds. We turned straight into it, barely managing to get the jib furled as the rain pelted us. I even glanced behind us to see if there was a chance of getting back out, but by then it had completely engulfed us. It felt as if the boat was actually inside the cloud itself.

For twenty minutes, the rain came down in sheets and the wind continued to howl. Then finally I could see a star in the sky ahead of us and knew that we must be coming out of it. Within seconds the rain and wind stopped. The storm had been so localized that waves hadn't even formed and the sea was still flat. The rest of the night the sky repeatedly alternated between perfectly clear and full of storm clouds.

Just before sunrise we went from six-thousand-feet deep seas to just forty almost instantly. We were officially back in the Bahamas. A few hours later we were anchored in six feet of crystal clear, emerald green water with not another boat in sight.

APRIL 9, 2007: EN ROUTE HOME

I had a big day of scraping yesterday. After just two weeks in the Luperón swamp, the boat had grown so much crap on the bottom that it was surprising that we were able to move at all. It took me three sessions to get it all off.

Jobs like that are made much easier in the beautiful waters of the Bahamas though. One thing I've often missed around the world has been anchoring in the ridiculously shallow waters that are so prevalent here. I could just about scrape the boat while standing up.

We have definitely come to the end of this sailing adventure. One look in the cupboards tells the story. Here is a complete rundown of the food we have got left. Four packs of Ramen from Florida, one can of tuna from the Galapagos, one soup from New Zealand, a can of curry from Australia, meatballs from Turkey, a few noodles, and a bag of Doritos from the Dominican Republic. That's every last morsel.

We bypassed all the good food in Puerto Rico in our dogged determination to eat everything on the boat and it looks like we might just do it. Sitting around after eating our can of soup tonight, I posed the question, "When are we ever going to cook again?" Actually, using the word *we* is overstating my involvement in the process by a long shot. Not to mention using the word cook. We both thought that over for a minute and came to the conclusion that once we reach Florida it is entirely possible we will never cook another meal in our lives. At least at the moment that is the goal.

Earlier that morning we had been awakened at five a.m. by the sound of a helicopter hovering over the boat. We both just laid there in bed as if we didn't hear a thing, too tired to go up and have a look. The chopper must have hovered there for a good five minutes, no doubt trying to call us on the VHF and wondering why nobody was coming out on deck. But we didn't move.

A couple of hours later after waking up I asked Ali, "Did you hear that helicopter?"

"Yeah it was annoying."

"But you didn't get up?" I asked.

"*You* didn't get up."

"Good point. I wonder what they wanted?"

This morning nobody rudely interrupted our sleep and after waking up refreshed we took off on our last passage for home. It was a beautiful day, with light winds and following seas. It was made even better because we were sailing over the Great Bahama Bank, with waters that never climbed over twenty-five feet deep. The ride is made much more interesting when we can lie up front and watch the fish and coral flow past beneath us.

APRIL 11, 2007: EN ROUTE HOME

Yesterday morning I was goofing around trying to get a cool picture of the boat under sail. The color of the water in the Bahamas is incredible and I'm sure we looked pretty awesome sailing across it, but since I didn't have a helicopter handy, I instead just reached way out over the edge of the boat with the camera. I got a pretty cool picture but also got caught by a splashing wave. Within one minute the camera had stopped working. That makes four digital cameras on this trip. Broken down as a monthly cost this makes our camera expense come out to $35 per month. Not exactly a monthly expense we anticipated before setting out.

The weather took an ugly turn last night. Immediately after dark the sky lit up with lightning. It was wicked stuff. Occasionally the lightning would strike vertically to the water, but more often it was horizontal and stretched for miles and miles across the horizon in a split second. It all seemed to emanate from one central core, like one of those mad scientist balls that makes your hair stand on end.

That core was directly in our path. We turned about forty degrees off course figuring we'd skirt by it within a half an hour or so. The wind was twenty knots coming from our right and the lightning storm was to our left. It seemed logical that we'd pass by it as it blew away from us. It didn't. Instead it seemed to parallel our track, gradually growing closer, and keeping us from getting any sleep. Around three a.m. it started breaking down, and the six-hour fireworks grand finale was finally over.

I woke up a few hours later expecting more downwind sailing fun for our last full day of sailing. Instead I came up and found Ali just shaking her head at me. She was not happy. I went outside to have a look and saw why. The wind was twenty knots and right on our nose. I looked up at the sky around us and saw nothing but a solid wall of blackness. The storms weren't over yet.

We soon had thirty-five knots howling through the rigging and kicking up awful, short, choppy seas. With just a bit of jib out we kept sailing, although way off course. Around noon it was still pouring rain. We couldn't see more than a hundred yards into the distance, but the wind had finally begun to die down.

The problem was that with the light winds and the left-over rough seas, we weren't able to make any progress towards home. Seeing as we were still sailing in water fifteen feet deep we did the sensible thing and dropped the anchor. The wind steadily decreased to zero, the seas flattened out, and within two hours we fired up the engine and got back underway.

Just one hundred miles to go and we've finally got our following seas back, with ten knots of wind, and three hours of shallow water left before hitting the Gulf Stream for our sleigh ride up the coast of Florida to Fort Lauderdale.

A COUPLE HOURS LATER the wind has picked up again and we are now galloping along. We were just visited by some very playful dolphins. We don't usually see them when conditions are rougher like this, more often they seem to show up when we are motoring in calm seas. Today they all raced from one wave to the next, surfing inside of it and then spinning and jumping out the back side. I'd say this is the thing that we will miss the most about life on a boat.

APRIL 13, 2007: FORT LAUDERDALE, FLORIDA

It's hard to believe but we've had two of the worst storms of our entire trip in just this last week. Today's takes the cake though, and is officially number one.

This morning was so calm that I slept in an hour later, which is unusual because our bodies have become like three-hour alarm clocks over the years on watch. When I came up I found that Ali had the whole house wide open with everything hanging out in the sun drying. It was an absolutely beautiful morning.

Two hours later we were ten miles off the coast of Miami when a black line appeared across the horizon. The lightning began as it slowly grew closer. We dropped the mainsail as a precaution and were sailing with the jib in very light winds, yet still flying along thanks to the Gulf Stream current.

As it started to rain I donned the raincoat and stood up at the captain's chair to keep an eye on the storm. Just then a bolt of lightning hit so close to us that the explosion almost seemed to precede the flash. I jumped down into the cockpit, and as I did there was suddenly a lot of noise up front as the wind had clocked around causing the jib to start flapping. Ali and I quickly got that sail furled and fired up both engines.

Within a minute the full force of the storm was upon us. The wind jumped to fifty knots, something we had only seen one other time, back in the Red Sea. The power was absolutely amazing. It felt as if we were caught inside a tornado. Not a hurricane, because let's face it, it wasn't that bad.

I kept the boat pointed straight into the wind while standing outside trying to keep watch. It was raining so hard that I had to turn my head every few seconds to spit out water and take a breath. Ali was standing in the doorway and was as scared as I've ever seen her.

"Are we okay?" she kept asking me over and over again with a trembling voice.

"We're fine, I promise," I kept reassuring her while not really sure myself.

Ali grabbed the VHF and immediately heard Maydays going out over the airwaves. The storm had apparently caught everybody off guard. We continued to hold our position, figuring this couldn't last too long. All we had to do was keep ourselves pointed into it and we'd come out the backside soon enough. Meanwhile things were getting frantic on the radio. A boat had been flipped over about twenty miles south of us and the Coast Guard was scrambling to coordinate a helicopter and ship to perform a search for a person who had washed overboard.

After what felt like days, the wind started to drop and we began to make our way towards the coast, ready to bail out to Miami if conditions didn't improve. By the time we were within view of the beaches, the sky was brightening and the wind had almost completely disappeared. We turned north again for Fort Lauderdale and two hours later were basking in the sunshine enjoying a beautiful afternoon.

WE PULLED INTO FORT LAUDERDALE at around five o'clock, and as a welcome home, we were almost immediately pulled over by some sort of water sheriff. He came up alongside and asked, just like a cruiser, if this was our boat. We said yes, and he then asked if we had an Illinois driver's license, rambling on about how Illinois required registration of its boats and yet he didn't see any registration stickers on us.

I didn't know what he was driving at but found it hard to believe that he had the authority to enforce Illinois State law down here. Ali came outside with our driver's licenses, at which point he almost seemed disappointed. He explained to us that there are a lot of tax cheats in Florida and then zoomed off. Apparently he had thought he was about to nab himself a real white collar criminal.

We arrived at the marina at 5:20, but being a city marina the employees had disappeared promptly at five. We grabbed a mooring nearby, put the dinghy in the water and headed for shore to celebrate.

First we had to make a call to customs. They seemed genuinely shocked that our last port was the Dominican Republic. "You sailed all the way from there?" I know, I thought, that is so far to sail a boat.

He asked for our address and phone number but seemed confused by those answers as well. "So you just live on your boat?"

I don't know if this guy was new to the job or what. He made us feel as if we were the first couple to ever sail into Fort Lauderdale. Eventually he issued us a twenty-four hour shore pass, but I think he may have red-flagged us as well. Something seemed fishy about these sailors.

Nothing appeared to have changed around the marina since the last time we'd been there over three years earlier. We walked to the very same restaurant that we had gone to the day we bought *Bumfuzzle*. It seemed like a fitting end to the trip. We ordered steaks, some really good beer, and talked about just how normal everything, including ourselves, suddenly felt.

APRIL 24, 2007: FORT LAUDERDALE, FLORIDA
The other night I was up late working on the computer when I heard the bedroom door being slammed into, followed by Ali racing up the stairs and flinging open the sliding doors to the cockpit.

"What the, what, where are, what, where are we, what was that?" She wasn't fully awake and had been dreaming that our anchor was dragging, despite the fact that we were in a marina slip and there was absolutely no wind. Since we have been living on a boat, Ali has not had a full night of sleep. She's always on edge just a little bit and wakes up throughout the night to go outside and check on everything. On the other hand I sleep like a baby through anything and everything, which drives her nuts.

APRIL 27, 2007: FORT LAUDERDALE, FLORIDA

We had sailed for years without insurance, but now back in the States we suddenly found that we needed it in order to sell the boat. None of the marinas would lift the boat out of the water if it wasn't insured. Going about the underwriting process was a wonderful experience.

"Hello, Boat America."

"Hi, I'm calling to check on the status of my application for insurance."

"Okay, let me check." Tap, tap, tap. "I'm sorry your application has been denied due to a lack of boating experience."

"Seriously? We just sailed around the world."

"Yes, but it says here that your prior boating experience was limited to an aluminum bass fishing boat."

"Yeah, prior to living on this boat full time for nearly four years and sailing it around the world."

"Hmmm. So where is this boat coming from?"

"Our last port you mean? The Dominican Republic."

"That's outside of the U.S. right? Okay, since this boat has been out of the country I would need a current survey."

"But we just want liability insurance, what does it matter what the boat is worth if we don't want you to pay for it? Besides, the only reason I need insurance is in order to be able to get the boat hauled out for a survey."

"Yes, that is a bit of a problem. I'm sorry I really must have a current survey in order to insure your boat. And even then, with your lack of boating experience I really don't think we could issue you coverage. Unless, perhaps . . . have you taken any boater safety courses?"

"Thanks for your help." Click.

MAY 4, 2007: FORT LAUDERDALE, FLORIDA

We cannot believe the storms we have been experiencing here in Florida. A couple of nights back we got nailed at three a.m. with a huge thunderstorm that brought fifty knot winds and some wicked lightning. To say we are looking forward to living on land again and not giving a toss what the weather is doing would be an understatement. But being on a boat, we spent the last two mornings staring outside at the rock wall fifty feet away trying to determine at what point our mooring ball would break loose, sending us smashing into it.

Our mooring held, but sadly not everything on the boat came through the storm unscathed. The winds dealt a death blow to the old, gray man-overboard pole. It had never saved a life, and according to many it never would have. But that gray pole did a great job of hanging our flag.

MAY 10, 2007: FORT LAUDERDALE, FLORIDA

Today Ali and I called our friend, a boat broker, and told him he had the boat listing. Trying to arrange all of the things necessary to sell a boat is not for us. It's not as easy as selling a car, or even a house for that matter. There are just too many things to coordinate, especially for a couple who don't even own a cell phone. He said no problem, and by that afternoon we had *Bum* tied up at one of their docks. Best of all, he knows everyone at the marinas and is able to get them to waive the insurance requirement.

MAY 11, 2007: FORT LAUDERDALE, FLORIDA

This morning Ali and I were up at six a.m. washing *Bum* for the last time, Ali on the inside and me on the out. Soon we were saying our goodbyes, and by eight o'clock we were on the road pointed north.

One would expect this to be an emotional time, but we really didn't feel anything. *Bum* had taken us around the world, just like we knew she would the day we bought her. There was never any doubt in our mind that she could make it. For that matter, there was never a doubt that the two of us could make it either. We'd accomplished what we had set out to do. We had sailed around the world.

MAY 12, 2007: SOMEWHERE IN GEORGIA

Oh, who am I kidding about not being emotional about this. I woke up crying this morning. Not because I missed *Bum*, but because I missed my dinghy. Who was going to supply him with the super glue he needed to live? He didn't stand a chance. Sure, *Bum* would sail again. Maybe even go around the world a second time. But our dinghy was breathing its last breath.

The last words the broker spoke to us were haunting me. "Maybe we ought to take the dinghy off and hide it on the side of that shed over there."

Ol' dinghy had seen his last days on the water, and so had we.

We have been back for a year now. Back where exactly, I can't say. All over the place, really. For the first couple years of this voyage, our plan was always to simply settle back into a life in Chicago. Make the big bucks, catch a downswing in the housing market, have kids, and generally try to behave like normal thirty-something adults. But then we fell in love with traveling, and any plans for normalcy went out the porthole.

Florida wasn't even in our rearview mirror before the first step in our next adventure was underway. Ali and I were lying in bed in a musty Interstate-side motel room when we came across a 1958 Volkswagen Panelvan for sale on the internet. By the time we left that morning, the money had been wired and we were well on our way to living the wandering gypsy lifestyle.

We spent the summer in Minnesota visiting family. Our thirst for adventure didn't wane though, and we found ourselves entered in a cross-country vintage automobile race. We ran it in our 1965 Porsche that has been in my family ever since I was brought home from the hospital in the front seat of it. The race was a lot of fun, giving us a chance to see small-town America up close; and best of all, we won the Rookie Class and the prize money to go along with it.

By the fall our families were probably tiring of us, so we loaded up for the road. This time we were packing the VW bus with pretty much everything we owned and setting out to circle the globe again. It was weird to see how much we had changed in the past few years. When we lived in Chicago, we wanted it all. Stuff, I guess, is what we would call it now. Now, packing up the VW, one of our biggest joys is in not owning anything. No more stuff.

We are much simpler now. Life can be picked up and moved on a moment's notice and we like that. We also like the fact that any time we want to settle down and accumulate stuff again we can. Borders and expectations mean little to us now. As long as the two of us are happy together, wherever we happen to be, that's all that is important.

The bus covered a lot of ground those first few months, first up through Canada, then down the West Coast of the States. We entered Baja, Mexico and found a place that we could travel, camp, and live simply again. For a few months we bummed around Mexico surfing, lying on the beach, learning Spanish, and eating delicious fish tacos. To be honest we were a little surprised at just how well a life lived out of the inside of a VW bus suited us. After four years in a boat, the concept of personal space didn't even exist any more. We were happy and having fun, what could be better?

After awhile, it was time to head back north. We drove to the States to prepare for an around-the-world race. This time, the vintage auto rally was going from New York to Paris via China. It was going to be an exciting time. A little more structured than we were used to, but we had our eyes on the prize. Unfortunately the Chinese government pulled their permits at the last moment, and the race was cancelled.

Seeing as it was now springtime and we were in Oregon with nothing to do, we decided to settle down for a couple of months, take over my mom's office, and write this book while we waited for the warm weather to come to Alaska, our next destination.

As I type this out we are counting down the days until we depart again. We're not sure what we'll find in Alaska, but are looking forward to it, nonetheless. From there our plans are to find a ship going somewhere exotic, load the bus onboard, and continue our wandering ways.

This is our life for now, and we are happy with what it has become. We don't live by anyone else's rules, which sounds incredibly cliché; but when done properly, it is an amazingly freeing feeling. Someday we'll change again. We'll settle down. Or maybe we won't. Who knows? We loved our time cruising, but have said we wouldn't do it again. Then, occasionally cruising creeps back into our discussions. I suppose it could happen. Our kids might want to see what we're always jabbering on about, and we might just be ready for another go around. We shall see.

We've heard it said, "Ali and Pat may have been around the world, but they haven't been around the block." Maybe that's true. Maybe we haven't learned nearly as much as we think we have. If not, at least we feel different. We feel like we've learned a lot about how others live in this world, and we have made changes in our lives because of that. Changes made for the better, as far as we are concerned. We look back on our cruising as a monumental life-altering moment in our lives, and it is one that we wouldn't trade for anything.